DR BARBARA INSPIRED

15 Day Gut Cleanse

Transform Your Gut in Just 15 Days! Discover O'Neill's Secrets for Lasting Health

Blessing Winfrey

Acknowledgment and Disclaimer:

This book is a tribute to the inspiration I've received from Barbara O'Neill's holistic health philosophy. However, it's important to clarify that this work is entirely original, crafted in strict adherence to copyright laws, and is born from my personal research, experiences, and interpretation of health and well-being. While inspired by O'Neill's approach, the concepts, strategies, and advice herein do not bear her direct endorsement nor do they reflect her specific teachings.

This publication aims to honor the foundation laid by Barbara O'Neill in the realm of natural health, yet it introduces my distinct insights and interpretations on the subject. It is designed to serve as an informative guide for those embarking on a journey toward improved health, with O'Neill's work serving as an inspirational springboard rather than a direct source.

Please note, this book is neither affiliated with nor officially endorsed by Barbara O'Neill. It stands as a separate, independent piece, intended for informational purposes only, and not as a substitute for professional medical advice. Readers should always seek the counsel of qualified health professionals for personal health concerns.

Table of Contents

INTRODUCTION

Your body is betraying you. Every ache, every mood swing, every extra pound – your gut could be the culprit. But you're being kept in the dark. The food industry and Big Pharma, don't want you to know the truth that Barbara O'Neill revealed: your gut holds the key to unlocking the good health you deserve. This book isn't just a cleanse; it's your weapon to fight back...because if you don't, your body will pay the price.

Barbara O'Neill, the revolutionary gut health expert's groundbreaking research revealed the shocking truth: a messed-up gut isn't just uncomfortable, it's the root cause of countless chronic illnesses.

Inspired by the revolutionary work of Barbara O'Neill, I've spent years getting to the bottom of gut health. The truth is, those quick-fix cleanses and trendy probiotics aren't doing squat. Real, lasting gut health – the kind that transforms your entire life – takes a deeper approach. Trust me, you won't find this in some clickbait article or on Dr. Google. This book holds the key to restoring your gut microbiome, and it's the only path to lasting wellness.

I had people like you in mind when writing this book, to remind you that a healthy gut microbiome is your secret weapon to manifesting a healthy life, and it's within reach. Within this book is a 15-Day Gut Cleanse and it is your step-by-step plan to finally:

- **Uncover What's Wrecking Your Gut:** (It's the stuff you do every day without thinking twice)

- **The Gut-Boosting Truth:** (Science-backed solutions, not fads)

- **15-Day Reset:** (Exactly what to eat, how to move, and the small changes that make a huge difference)

Don't wait until it's too late. Every day you ignore your gut is another day you're robbing yourself of the energetic, healthy life you deserve. Let's face it, ignoring this problem won't make it go away; so here's your wake-up call!

WHO IS BARBARA O'NEILL?

Barbara O'Neill is a naturopath and natural health educator with a focus on gut health. She promotes a holistic approach, emphasizing dietary adjustments, herbal remedies, and lifestyle changes to restore gut balance.

Barbara O'Neill's Key Principles

- **Elimination Diet:** O'Neill advocates removing common allergens and irritants like gluten, dairy, and refined sugars. This can help identify food sensitivities that contribute to gut dysfunction.

- **Focus on Whole Foods:** Her approach prioritizes unprocessed, nutrient-dense foods such as fruits, vegetables, whole grains (if tolerated), and lean proteins.

- **Supplementation:** She recommends probiotics, prebiotics, digestive enzymes, and gut-healing nutrients like L-glutamine.

- **Stress Management:** O'Neill recognizes the gut-brain connection and suggests stress-reducing practices like yoga, meditation, or spending time in nature.

Barbara O'Neill's approach offers potential benefits to gut health, prioritizes a whole-food diet, manages stress, explores the wonders of your microbiome, and with the help of the secrets contained in this book, you can create a personalized plan for optimal gut and overall well-being.

PART 1:
IT ALL BEGINS IN YOUR GUT

CHAPTER 1

What is the Gut Microbiome?

"The gut is the seat of all feeling, the belly of the brain." - Emeran Mayer, MD

Forget what you think you know about your insides. Your gut isn't just a food processing plant; it's a crowded city of tons of bacteria, fungi, and other microscopic critters. This is your gut microbiome, and it's waging war inside you RIGHT NOW.

Think of it like this: you've got an army of good guys (the beneficial microbes) fighting to protect your health. But there's also a horde of bad guys (the harmful ones) constantly trying to break down your defenses. Junk food, stress, antibiotics... each of these is a weapon of mass destruction for your gut's good bacteria.

When the bad guys win, that's when the trouble starts. Chronic inflammation, a wrecked immune system, and even your risk for serious diseases like cancer and heart trouble skyrocket. This isn't just about feeling bloated; this is about your body slowly falling apart from the inside out.

You can take back control, but it starts with understanding your gut microbiome and learning how to boost those good bacteria. Because here's the thing – they're your secret superpower for unlocking the health you've been desperately chasing.

Ways to Boost the Good Bacteria Resident in Your Gut

Think popping a probiotic is the answer? Think again. Your gut is filled with countless number of bacteria, both good and bad. The goal isn't to just add more, it's to make an environment where the good guys thrive and multiply, naturally crowding out the troublemakers. Here's how to turn your gut into a prosperous place for beneficial bacteria:

1. **Feed Your Inner Army:** Prebiotics are the special fibers that your good bacteria feast on. Think of them as fertilizer for your gut garden. Load up on:

   o Garlic, onions, leeks (stinky, but powerful!)
   o Asparagus, Jerusalem artichokes, bananas

- Whole grains like oats and barley

2. **Ditch the Gut Wreckers:** Processed foods, sugar, and artificial sweeteners are like poison to your beneficial bacteria. They starve the good guys and feed the bad. Cut them out as much as possible, your gut will thank you.

3. **Go Fermented, Get Wild:** Fermented foods like sauerkraut, kimchi, yogurt, and kefir are teeming with live, active cultures that reinforce your gut's defenses. Aim for a small serving every day.

4. **The Polyphenol Power-Up:** These plant compounds act like elite gut protectors. Find them in:

  - Berries (blueberries, raspberries – the darker the better!)
  - Colorful veggies
  - Dark chocolate (yes, finally a good excuse!)

The Science behind harboring good bacteria in the Gut

This isn't just about better digestion. When your good bacteria flourish, you'll see:

- **Supercharged Immunity:** A strong gut = a strong defense against colds, flu, and more.

- **Mental Clarity:** That brain fog lifts as your gut-brain connection strengthens.

- **Effortless Energy:** When your body absorbs nutrients properly, you have fuel to burn.

- **Glowing Skin:** A healthy gut radiates from within, reducing inflammation and breakouts.

Don't expect overnight miracles, but commit to this way of life and you will see results. More energy, clearer skin, better digestion – the benefits ripple out into your whole life. Think of it as training an internal army to fight for your health, day in and day out.

CHAPTER 2

The Impact of Diet, Lifestyle, and the Environment on Gut Health

"Let food be thy medicine and medicine be thy food." – Hippocrates

Way back in ancient Greece, Hippocrates knew something we're finally rediscovering: What you put into your body has a profound impact on your overall health. And your gut? It's the epicenter of that impact.

Barbara O'Neill helps us understand just how deep this connection goes. Think of your gut as the foundation of a house. If it's crumbling, the whole thing becomes unstable, no matter how pretty the living room looks.

The Science Behind the Wreckage

So, what's wrecking your gut microbiome (that complex ecosystem of bacteria living in your gut)? Let's break it down:

- **The Standard American Diet (SAD):** Yes, I'm calling it out. Processed foods, refined sugar, unhealthy fats...this stuff isn't just making you gain weight. It's feeding the BAD bacteria in your gut, the kind that triggers inflammation, messes with your immunity and sets the stage for chronic diseases. It's like pouring gasoline on a fire.

- **Stress Overload:** When you're constantly in fight-or-flight mode (thanks, modern life!), your body shifts resources away from digestion. This messes with your gut bacteria balance, leaving you vulnerable to all sorts of problems. O'Neill taught us that chronic stress is like a gut punch – weakening your defenses over time.

- **Environmental Toxins:** They're everywhere – pesticides in food, chemicals in cleaning products, even the air we breathe. These toxins can damage the delicate lining of your gut, disrupt your microbiome, and open the door to inflammation throughout your body. Yuck.

- **Antibiotics and Other Meds:** Sometimes they're necessary lifesavers, but antibiotics wipe out good bacteria along with the bad. Other medications like acid blockers and NSAIDs (think ibuprofen) can also wreak gut havoc. Long-term use disrupts that vital bacterial balance.

- **Lack of Sleep:** When you skip sleep, it throws your entire body out of order, including your gut. Studies show that sleep deprivation can lead to an unhealthy microbiome, increasing your risk of obesity, and diabetes, you name it.

What Happens When Your Gut Goes Haywire

This isn't just about feeling bloated after a bad meal. A messed-up gut has ripple effects throughout your entire body:

- **Digestive Distress:** Obviously, things like gas, bloating, constipation, diarrhea...no fun. But this is often the first sign of a deeper imbalance.

- **Weakened Immunity:** A huge portion of your immune system lives in your gut! An unhealthy microbiome leaves you vulnerable to every bug going around, plus chronic inflammation that's at the root of many diseases.

- **Brain Fog and Mood Swings:** Your gut is your "second brain"! It produces neurotransmitters that impact your mood, focus, and even anxiety levels. O'Neill's work highlighted this gut-brain connection in a big way.

- **Skin Problems:** Acne, eczema, rashes...they can all be a sign that your gut is out of order. Inflammation in the gut often shows up on your skin.

- **Weight Gain and Metabolic Issues:** Your gut bacteria play a huge role in metabolism and how your body uses energy. An unbalanced gut can make it way harder to lose weight or keep it off.

- **Chronic Diseases:** The science is clear: long-term gut problems are linked to serious conditions like autoimmune disorders, heightened inflammation, a major driver of heart diseases, type 2 diabetes, and even some cancers.

Feeling Overwhelmed? Don't Panic!

Look, this might seem scary, but there's good news: Your gut is incredibly resilient. By giving it the right support, informed by O'Neill's revolutionary approach, you can take back control. Think of it as a system reset, a chance to build a healthier foundation from the inside out.

Reclaiming Your Gut Health the Barbara O'Neill Way

Here's where things get exciting. O'Neill wasn't about quick fixes or restrictive diets. She focused on sustainable, holistic changes that nourish your gut for the long haul:

- **Ditch the Processed Crap:** Focus on whole, unprocessed foods – veggies, fruits, healthy fats, and quality protein. Your gut bacteria will thank you.

- **Prioritize Probiotics and Prebiotics:** Probiotics are the good bacteria, and prebiotics are the fiber that feeds them. Think fermented foods like yogurt and sauerkraut, or a high-quality supplement.

- **Manage Stress Mindfully:** Easier said than done, I know! But techniques like meditation, yoga, or simply spending time in nature can make a huge difference for both your gut and your mind.

- **Be Mindful of Medications:** Work closely with your doctor to see if the medications you're on could be negatively impacting your gut health, and if there are alternatives.

- **Pay Attention to Your Environment:** Minimize exposure to toxins where possible. Choose natural cleaning products, filter your water, and consider an air purifier.

It's not a hopeless situation, although it might feel overwhelming. Your gut microbiome is resilient! Changing your diet, managing stress, and making smarter lifestyle choices can create a huge turnaround for your gut city. That's why a targeted reset with a cleanse program is needed to shift things into high gear.

CHAPTER 3

When Your Body Is Due For a Gut Cleanse

"The gut is not a pipe, but a living, breathing ecosystem that contains nearly 100 trillion microorganisms that affect our bodies in far more ways than scientists ever imagined." – Dr. David Perlmutter, Grain Brain

Your gut is astonishingly complex – part digestive system, part communication network, and a major hub of your immune system. Within this complex system are microorganisms that directly impact everything from your weight to your moods. This world within, your gut microbiome, is essential for good health. But when it becomes overrun by unhealthy bacteria, yeast, parasites, or even superbugs, everything is thrown off balance. Think of it this way: if your body is like a flourishing garden, these harmful invaders are like voracious weeds. They steal nutrients, damage beneficial organisms, and release toxins that wreak havoc far beyond the gut.

This chapter will help you identify when your body is signaling that a gut cleanse is in order. We'll also explore the four Colon Corruptors that contribute to this disruption, and how the 15-Day Gut Cleanse works and I'll share strategies and insights to help you restore balance and reclaim vibrant health.

The Four Colon Corruptors

Corruptor #1: Overgrowth of Yeast

Yeast normally exists in small amounts in various parts of the body. But when it proliferates in the gut, it leads to a condition called candidiasis. Yeast has a sweet tooth, and overconsumption of sugar, refined grains, or even some fruits can fuel its growth. Symptoms of yeast overgrowth extend far beyond the gut, and may include:

- Fatigue, headaches, brain fog
- Bloating, gas, indigestion
- Sugar cravings, mood swings
- Skin issues like acne and rashes
- Immune system dysfunction

Corruptor #2: Parasitic Infestation

Parasites are living organisms that can set up shop in your gut, feeding off you and your nutrients. Although images of parasites often evoke faraway countries, it's startlingly common in the developed world as well. Contamination of water or produce, as well as contact with pets, can increase your risk. Common symptoms include:

- Chronic fatigue, unexplained weakness
- Digestive issues like diarrhea and constipation
- Skin issues, itchy rashes
- Weight fluctuations, difficulty losing weight
- Insomnia, grinding teeth at night

Corruptor #3: Superbugs

Superbugs are bacteria that have become resistant to most antibiotics. Overuse of antibiotics has contributed to their alarming rise, and they can cause serious, sometimes life-threatening infections. Superbugs like MRSA (methicillin-resistant *Staphylococcus aureus*) and *H. pylori* can wreak havoc on the gut, leading to:

- Stomach ulcers
- Diarrhea, nausea, inflammation
- Increased risk of various chronic diseases

Corruptor #4: Food Sensitivities

Unlike true allergies, which trigger immediate reactions, food sensitivities manifest slowly. It may take hours or even days for symptoms to appear. Common culprits include gluten, dairy, corn, and soy. These sensitivities disrupt gut balance, and may cause:

- Digestive upset - bloating, gas, constipation, diarrhea
- Unexplained headaches, joint pain, skin issues
- Brain fog, mood swings, fatigue
- Difficulty losing weight

When Your Body Signals the Need for a Cleanse

If you're experiencing any combination of the symptoms described above, your body is likely crying out for help. Here are some additional signs to watch for:

- **Persistent Digestive woes:** Chronic constipation, bloating, gas, and diarrhea are signs your gut is struggling.

- **Skin problems:** Skin conditions like acne, eczema, and psoriasis often reflect internal imbalances.

- **Brain fog:** Difficulty focusing, trouble remembering things, and poor mood may indicate inflammation and toxins affecting your brain.

- **Constant fatigue:** Your gut is a major energy producer, and when it's out of whack, you'll feel it.

The Gut Cleanse Solution

My 15-Day Gut Cleanse is a three-stage plan – *Reinforce, Cleanse, and Replenish (**RCR**)* – designed to help you eliminate the four Colon Corruptors, rebuild beneficial bacteria, and restore your health. Here's a preview of some key strategies:

- **Anti-inflammatory Nutrition:** Avoiding processed foods, refined carbs, and excess sugar starves harmful invaders. Focus on whole, nourishing foods.

- **Gut-healing Supplements:** Probiotics flood your gut with beneficial bacteria, while specific herbal blends and supplements target yeast, parasites, and superbugs.

- **Lifestyle Support:** Stress reduction, adequate sleep, and gentle exercise further boost your body's healing system.

When those signals of imbalance become undeniable, a cleanse is the way to support your body in flushing out the troublemakers, strengthening its defenses, and restoring that vibrant feeling of health.

How the 15-Day Gut Cleanse works

It's easy to blame our health problems on germs, but the truth is they're not always the root cause. Think of your gut as a battlefield. If the terrain is healthy and balanced, invading germs will struggle to survive. But if it's weakened – hello, sickness! The Gut Flush Plan is all about making your gut an inhospitable place for bad bugs.

In the previous section, we spoke about the three steps for an effective Gut cleanse which are **REINFORCE (Day 1-5), CLEANSE (Day 6-10), AND REPLENISH (Day 11-15)**. Let's talk more below;

1. REINFORCE

Sweet Sabotage: Sugar and Your Gut

Sugar is the ultimate bad guy for your gut. Here's why:

- **Party Time for Parasites and Yeast:** They love to munch on sugar and multiply quickly. This leads to bloating, gas, and feeling generally awful.

- **Artificial Sweeteners Are No Better:** Studies show many of us struggle to digest them, further messing with our guts.

- **Moldy Foods are a No-Go:** Many foods, particularly those including yeast (cheese, mushrooms, etc.), can add to the yeast overgrowth in your system.

Step 1: Strengthen Your Gut Defenses

The first stage of the Gut Cleanse Plan is all about strengthening your gut's defenses against those troublesome Colon Corruptors. Here's the plan of attack:

- **Eliminate the Sweets:** This means no sugars, including fruit and artificial sweeteners, for the first two weeks of the plan. The Gut Flush substitute, Flora-Key, is an exception thanks to its prebiotic powers (more on that later).

- **Power Up with Probiotics & Prebiotics:** Think of probiotics as your gut's good bacteria army. Here's how to boost them:

- **Probiotic Foods:** Include at least one daily (think yogurt, sauerkraut, and miso).

- **Prebiotic Foods:** These are like food for your probiotics! Aim for TWO servings daily (think onions, garlic, Jerusalem artichokes).

- **Soluble Fiber is Your Friend:** This type dissolves in water and feeds your good bacteria. Include at least two servings of soluble fiber foods daily (think seeds, nuts, oatmeal).

- **The Power of Omegas:** Omega-3 fatty acids, found in fish and flaxseed oil, have a bonus benefit of helping your gut fight infection. Include fish at least twice a week and flaxseed oil daily.

- **Hydration is Key:** Water keeps your system running smoothly and makes it harder for bugs to settle in. Aim to drink half your body weight in ounces each day.

- **Strengthen with Salt:** It may sound strange, but salt is a natural preservative that can help fight bad bacteria. Aim for a teaspoon spread across meals throughout the day.

- **Say Goodbye to Coffee (Temporarily):** Coffee can contribute to constipation and mess with your gut flora. During Week One, switch to alternative teas like chicory or dandelion.

- **Ditch the Alcohol:** Alcohol is a major gut irritant and weakens your terrain. Consider taking a break while doing the Gut Flush Plan.

So, to simplify, it's all about cutting out things that make your gut a party zone for bad bugs (sugar, moldy foods) and replacing them with things that strengthen your gut's defenses (probiotics, prebiotics, good fats). It's like a supercharged spring cleaning for your insides!

2. CLEANSE

Cleaning out those Colon Corruptors

Okay, so we have successfully reinforced our gut against the nasty things that can mess it up – the Colon Corruptors. Those are things like sugar, yeast, bad bacteria, and the whole gang. Now, we're kicking those invaders out with a super deep clean! It's like spring cleaning for your insides.

The Importance of Cleansing

Imagine the Colon Corruptors have been hanging out way too long, eating all your good food, and causing commotion. We need to show them their way out.

This 'Gut Cleanse' is all about using powerful foods, herbs, spices, and special tactics to show them the door. We're going to make their environment so unfriendly, they'll pack up and leave voluntarily.

Gut Cleanse Tactics

Let's dive into the awesome strategies we'll be using to cleanse your system:

Tactic #1: Bet on Beta-carotene

You know how carrots, squash, and sweet potatoes are all bright orange or yellow? That's beta-carotene! This stuff is a powerhouse for your body. Think of it as the raw material your body turns into vitamin A, which is awesome for your immune system, eyes, and more. Plus, it specifically protects your intestines. It's like putting up armor plates along your digestive tract.

Tactic #2: Go Coconutty!

Okay, we're ditching the olive oil this week and switching to coconut oil. The special fats inside, especially lauric acid, are like tiny warriors against bacteria, viruses, yeast...all the bad guys. Coconut oil is so powerful against pathogens that people have been using it to stay healthy for thousands of years!

Tactic #3: Keep Out the Unfriendly Carbs

Remember, sugars and even some 'good' starches can still feed yeast and parasites. So, we're moderating those for a bit. Don't worry, you'll still get some gluten-free grains and starchy veggies. And if you have super sensitive digestion, we'll tweak things even more, following something called the Specific Carbohydrate Diet. That's all about keeping carbs very simple to make digestion extra easy.

Tactic #4: Spice up Your Life

Cinnamon, garlic, oregano, and cayenne – these are our weapons this week! They're like little superheroes against bacteria – the ones that cause food poisoning, ulcers, and all that nasty stuff. Plus, they have a ton of other health benefits. Get ready for some seriously flavorful food!

Tactic #5: More Colon Corruptor Killer Foods

We're bringing in some extra special foods this week – pumpkin seeds, kelp, sauerkraut, almonds, and radishes. These foods might sound a little unusual, but they have natural compounds that parasites and other troublemakers *hate*. Plus, they're packed with other healthy stuff too.

Tactic #6: Add Cleansing Beverages

Hydrating properly is key for flushing your system. On top of your water, we're adding Pau d'Arco and mugwort teas. Pau d'Arco is like a rainforest superhero – it fights bacteria, viruses, fungus, you name it. Mugwort's have been used for ages to get rid of worms. Think of them as your internal cleaning crew!

Colon Cleansing Power-Ups

We need to get colonics or do enemas. It's a little intense, but basically, the idea is deep cleaning your intestines with water and sometimes additives. You can think of it as a supercharged way to wash away toxins and anything else hanging around too long. It's an option to boost your cleansing process.

Why All the Fuss?

Our mission in Week Two is to get your gut sparkling clean by showing those Colon Corruptors the door. They wreak havoc and cause bloating, tiredness, and all sorts of issues. With a good internal cleanse, you might be amazed at how much better you feel, and how much clearer your mind is. Get ready for a serious energy boost!

Benefits of some foods that aid Gut Cleansing

- **Cinnamon:** Helps to control blood sugar!

- **Garlic:** Not only great against bad guys, it might help keep nasty antibiotic-resistant bugs at bay.

- **Cayenne pepper:** This spice helps fight cancer cells and protect against food poisoning. It's like a fire extinguisher for your insides!

- **Pumpkin seeds:** Packed with antioxidants that keep your digestive system healthy, and even help your prostate if you're a guy.

- **Kelp:** Helps your body fight infections and may even lower your risk of certain cancers. Seaweed to the rescue!

- **Sauerkraut:** it has anti-cancer properties.

- **Almonds:** Not only great for parasites, but they keep your arteries clear and reduce heart problems.

- **Radishes:** helps fight the Candida fungus, plus they stimulate your liver functions.

This is just the beginning of a 3-week journey! Think of these two weeks as 'spring cleaning.' You've got rid of the junk food (Reinforce) and now you're flushing toxins and bad microbes out the door. Pretty soon, we'll move into actually healing your digestive system to make it stronger than ever.

3. REPLENISH

Week Three: Replenish Your Gut

So, you've successfully reinforced your gut and cleaned out a bunch of bad stuff. Now, it's time to feed your body with healthy, nourishing foods. Week three is where things start to feel like a sustainable way of eating for life!

The goal for this week is still to keep up the good habits you've built – boosting those good bacteria, kicking out the colon corruptors, and helping your gut lining heal. But you'll also build a foundation of healthy eating habits for the long haul.

Why Week Three is Important

Okay, let's be honest, eliminating things like fruits and starches for a couple of weeks was tough. But we did it to starve out the bad stuff in your gut. Now that you've built up your defenses a little, we can start adding some of those tasty things back in... Carefully. The idea is to keep doing all the good things we've been doing but with a wider variety of foods.

Think of it like building a house. You wouldn't skip the foundation work and start putting on a fancy roof, right? Same with your gut – we have to make sure the base is strong and healthy before we can enjoy all the good things without risking problems later.

The Replenish Tactics: How to Promote Gut Health

Five key ideas centered on replenishing your gut in this week:

1. **Protein is Power:** Did you know that your gut is *made* of protein? It's basically like the bricks that form your intestinal walls. Eating protein doesn't just build muscle– it helps repair your gut lining, keeping things strong and less likely to get inflamed. Plus, protein keeps those good-for-digestion smooth muscles healthy. Yes, protein is especially good, but you'll also get plenty from lean meat, fish, and eggs.

2. **Veg Out**: Too much protein without veggies is a no-go. Not only do veggies make you feel full and satisfied, but they're packed with nutrients and natural stuff that

protects you from food poisoning! Think of those colorful vegetables as little armies fighting the bad guys in your gut.

3. **Sweet Success (with limits)**: We cut out fruits earlier to starve out the yeast, but now you can add some back! While they have sugar, fruits are also loaded with good antioxidants and fiber. Think of them as a natural boost for your immune system. This week you can rotate a couple of fruits into your day – think apples, berries, or citrus.

4. **Starches Are Back** (Kind Of): Beans, my friend, are your new staple. Protein? Check. Fiber? Check. Awesome to help those good bacteria? Check! Those guys produce butyrate – it's like a magic potion that helps your gut heal and function at its best. They're a little tougher to digest at first, so build up to them slowly.

5. **Plus Some Extras**: Slippery elm tea will be your new favorite beverage – it's super soothing, like a warm blanket for your insides. And the supplements, L-glutamine and DGL, are like superheroes specifically for gut repair.

Wait, Isn't Coffee... Bad?

Okay, we need to chat about coffee enemas. I know it sounds weird, but it's a different story than drinking it. Think of it as a detox for your liver and gallbladder, which in turn helps clean out your colon. Honestly, it's a powerful deep cleanse for your system.

In conclusion, the Gut Cleanse plan is all about balance. Yes, we're fighting off the bad stuff, but just as importantly, we're building the good backup. It's really about nourishing your body so it can heal and thrive.

This is a way to permanently change your relationship with food. Think of these three weeks as a stepping stone to long-term health, not a sprint to the finish line. We're in this for the long haul!

Before you run off to the next chapter, let's get a bit practical...

Here's a quick rundown of some new (and returning) foods allowed in the replenishing stage of the plan:

- Protein power: Aim for about 8 ounces of lean meats a day, a couple of eggs, and keep those whey protein shakes coming.

- Veggie bonanza: Get creative with those veggies! Think of at least five servings of those colorful, non-starchy veggies a day.

- Fruit is back: Add a couple of servings – apples, berries, plums, you get the idea. Spread them out throughout the day.

- Hello, beans: Think black beans, lentils, and garbanzos – they're super healthy, just go easy at first if you're not used to them.

- Tea time: Get those capsules of slippery elm and make it a tea – aim for a couple of cups a day.

Don't forget those supplements either. L-glutamine is like a multivitamin for your gut lining and DGL helps heal any damage down there.

Common Gut Issues and Their Symptoms

We often wait for some magic pill instead of tapping into our body's natural healing power. Barbara O'Neill understood this. Gut disorders aren't just a nuisance – they're the first sign your body is screaming for help.

Revealing the Gut-Health Saboteurs

Here are the common issues and what they might be trying to tell you:

1. **The Bloat That Won't Quit:** Feeling like a pufferfish after meals isn't just uncomfortable, it's a major red flag. The gas buildup could be from what you eat, but also food intolerances, an imbalance of those good gut bacteria O'Neill talked about, or even low stomach acid (yes, that's important for digestion too!).

2. **Bathroom Troubles: Constipation vs. Diarrhea:** Both are brutal. Constipation is like a traffic jam in your intestines...toxins build up instead of exiting efficiently. Diarrhea is the opposite extreme, with your body flushing out nutrients before they can be used. Diet is a factor, but so is stress (our gut is like our 'second brain'), infections, and even gut flora imbalances.

3. **Heartburn, Reflux, the Burning Fire:** You know the feeling...that fiery acid creeping up your throat. It's NOT just from spicy food. This is your stomach acid going rogue due to stress, certain medications, or issues like a hiatal hernia (it's surprisingly common). Left unchecked, it can cause way more problems than just discomfort.

4. **The Energy Drain and Brain Fog:** Ever feel exhausted even after sleeping? Struggle to focus? Your gut might be partly to blame. When your gut isn't working right, nutrient absorption goes haywire, starving your brain and body of the fuel they need.

5. **Cranky Moods and Low Spirits:** Did you know 90% of your serotonin – that 'feel-good' chemical – is made in your gut? Healthy gut bacteria play a huge role in regulating mood. An inflamed gut? Well, that can lead to anxiety, irritability, and even depression in some cases.

6. Skin Freak-Outs Acne, eczema, rashes... these aren't just unlucky genes. Often, your gut is screaming through your skin. Inflammation, toxins that can't escape, all of it shows up eventually. O'Neill hammered home this gut-skin connection.

Unchecked Gut Dysfunction gets worse

This is Just the Beginning...Think of these as those flashing warning signs on your car dashboard:

- **Leaky Gut:** Sounds gross, is gross. Your gut lining is supposed to be selective. When it's damaged (bad diet, stress!), larger food particles and toxins leak into your bloodstream, causing chronic inflammation, the root of many nasty diseases.

- **Weakened Immunity:** 70% of your immune system is headquartered in your gut! A messed-up microbiome equals a lousy defense against every bug that comes along. Ever feel like you catch everything? Time to fix your gut.

- **Autoimmune Disorders:** Leaky gut, bad bacteria, all of it can trigger your immune system to go haywire and start attacking your own body. Conditions like rheumatoid arthritis, Hashimoto's, and even Type 1 Diabetes are increasingly linked to gut health.

The Science-Backed Truth

Okay, that was a lot of doom and gloom. But here's the good news: So much of this is reversible, and O'Neill made understanding these mechanisms easier. Here's the science simplified:

- **It's ALL About the Microbiome:** Your gut is home to a countless number of bacteria, fungi, and other microbes. It's like a rainforest ecosystem. These guys are key to digestion, immunity, and even mental health. When the beneficial ones are outnumbered by the bad guys...health crumbles.

- **Inflammation: The Enemy Within:** This isn't just a swollen ankle. Chronic low-grade inflammation, often stemming from the gut, is the silent killer at the root of heart disease, cancer, and Alzheimer's...the big ones.

- **It's Not JUST What You Eat:** Yes, diet matters massively. But O'Neill taught us to think holistically: stress, sleep, how you move your body, toxins you're exposed to... all of it impacts your gut, for better or worse.

Healing your gut takes time and personalization. But, once you start feeling those results...more energy, better mood, clearer skin...you'll never want to go back to your old ways!

PART 1 EXERCISE

Fun Gut Health Quiz

As you learned in the chapter, our gut health is crucial for our overall well-being. It can impact everything from our digestion and mood to our skin health and even our risk of chronic diseases.

But how much do you know about your gut? Take this fun quiz to find out!

Instructions:

1. Read each question carefully.

2. Choose the answer that you think is best.

3. No peeking at the answers!

4. Once you've finished the quiz, scroll down to the bottom to check your answers and learn more about gut health.

Ready? Let's begin!

Question 1: What is the gut microbiome?

- **A:** A type of stomach acid

- **B:** The network of neurons in your intestines

- **C:** A collection of trillions of microorganisms living in your gut

Question 2: Which of the following foods is an excellent source of prebiotics?

- **A:** Garlic

- **B:** Steak

- **C:** White bread

Question 3: Your gut is often referred to as your "second brain." Why?

- **A:** It produces neurotransmitters that affect mood and focus

- **B:** It stores memories and experiences from your past

- **C:** It has the power to override decisions made by your actual brain

Question 4: Chronic stress can have a negative impact on your gut health.

- **A:** True

- **B:** False

Question 5: What is one key benefit of having a healthy gut microbiome?

- **A:** Stronger immune system
- **B:** Easier weight loss
- **C:** Improved sleep quality
- **D:** All of the above

Question 6: Which of the following is NOT a common cause of an unhealthy gut?

- **A:** Lack of sleep
- **B:** Daily exercise
- **C:** Antibiotic overuse

Question 7: Probiotics are:

- **A:** Harmful bacteria
- **B:** Live, beneficial bacteria
- **C:** A type of digestive enzyme

Question 8: Which of the following is a sign of a potential gut imbalance?

- **A:** Persistent bloating
- **B:** Regular bowel movements
- **C:** Clear, glowing skin

Question 9: Fermented foods like yogurt, kimchi, and sauerkraut are excellent for gut health because they...

- **A:** Are low in calories
- **B:** Are high in fiber and probiotics
- **C:** Help curb your appetite

Question 10: What does the term "colon corruptors" refer to?

- **A:** Substances that disrupt the balance of your gut microbiome
- **B:** Types of healthy bacteria living in the colon
- **C:** Ingredients that trigger bloating

Question 11: Which beverage is recommended during the Cleanse stage of the 15-Day Gut Cleanse?

- **A:** Coffee
- **B:** Pau d'Arco Tea

- **C:** Green Smoothies

Question 12: What is the main purpose of a gut cleanse?

- **A:** To eliminate toxins and harmful organisms from the digestive system
- **B:** To permanently eliminate all unhealthy cravings
- **C:** To cure all digestive problems for good

Question 13: Why are pumpkin seeds beneficial for gut health?

- **A:** They contain natural compounds that may help fight parasites
- **B:** They're high in vitamin C which boosts the immune system
- **C:** They're an excellent source of magnesium

Question 14: The Replenish stage of the Gut Cleanse focuses on:

- **A:** Reintroducing healthy foods to support long-term gut health
- **B:** Eliminating all sugars for good
- **C:** Continuing strict dietary restrictions

Question 15: Leaky gut refers to

- **A:** A normal function of the digestive system
- **B:** The feeling of fullness after a large meal
- **C:** A compromised gut lining that allows toxins into the bloodstream

Question 16: True or False: Taking a probiotic supplement is the best and only way to improve your gut health.

- **A:** True
- **B:** False

Question 17: Cinnamon, garlic, and cayenne pepper are considered beneficial during a gut cleanse because:

- **A:** They taste delicious
- **B:** They have natural antimicrobial properties
- **C:** They enhance the flavor of bland foods

Question 18: A gut cleanse should be viewed as:

- **A:** A quick fix for weight loss
- **B:** A reset to kickstart healthy habits

- **C:** A long-term, sustainable diet

Question 19: Which of the following is NOT a common symptom of Candida overgrowth?

- **A:** Persistent fatigue
- **B:** Improved concentration
- **C:** Sugar cravings

Question 20: Good gut health has been linked to a lower risk of:

- **A:** Type 2 Diabetes
- **B:** Autoimmune disorders
- **C:** Heart disease
- **D:** All of the above

Answer Key

1. C
2. A
3. A
4. A
5. D
6. B
7. B
8. A
9. B
10. A
11. B
12. A
13. A
14. A
15. C
16. B
17. B

18. B

19. B

20. D

How did you do?

- **15 correct answers:** You're a gut health champion! You clearly understand the importance of gut health and how to keep your gut bacteria happy.

- **8-10 correct answers:** You're on the right track! Keep learning about gut health and making small changes to improve your gut bacteria balance.

- **3-6 correct answers:** Don't worry, everyone starts somewhere! This quiz is a great starting point to learn more about gut health and how to improve yours.

Want to learn more?

Part 1 offers a great resource for understanding the basics of gut health.

Remember, taking care of your gut is an investment in your overall health and well-being. By making small changes to your diet, lifestyle, and habits, you can support your gut health and reap the many benefits it has to offer.

PART 2: NOURISHING YOUR GUT FOR OPTIMAL HEALTH

CHAPTER 4

The Power of a Balanced Diet

"If you keep good food in your fridge, you'll eat good food."- Errick McAdams

Okay, forget everything you thought you knew about "dieting." This isn't about starvation or cutting out whole food groups. This is about giving your body the tools to heal itself from the inside out. Think of it like pressing the reset button on your health.

A balanced diet has become such a buzzword that sometimes it loses all meaning. Trust me, I get it. You're bombarded with conflicting advice, and fad diets promising miracle solutions, and it's enough to make anyone throw up their hands and order takeout.

But here's the deal that many "wellness gurus" conveniently forget: True, lasting health isn't about deprivation or some crazy restrictive plan. And, as Barbara O'Neill emphasized, it all starts with the gut. Let's break down why a balanced diet is the foundation of your gut cleanse success – and beyond:

1. **Your Gut: Not Just About Digestion**

Think of your gut as the CEO of your body. It doesn't just process food; it impacts:

- **Your Immune System:** A whopping 70% of your immune cells live in that gut lining! A healthy gut microbiome (the community of bacteria) acts like a shield, protecting you from getting sick all the time.

- **Your Brain:** Ever heard of the gut-brain axis? Turns out, your gut bacteria produce neurotransmitters that affect mood, anxiety, and even your ability to focus.

- **Your Metabolism:** A sluggish gut can mess with hormones that control hunger, fat storage, and how effectively you burn calories.

- **Your Skin:** Surprise! Gut inflammation often shows up as breakouts, eczema, and uneven tone - basically, your skin not looking its best.

2. **What DOES a Balanced Diet Look Like for Gut Health?**

Forget calorie counting or obsessing over a single macronutrient. Think of food as the way to nurture your gut, and in return, your gut nurtures the rest of you. Here's what that means:

- **Whole Foods FTW:** Ditch the processed junk! Think colorful fruits and veggies, whole grains, lean protein, and healthy fats (avocados, nuts, oily fish). This delivers the fiber and nutrients your good gut bacteria crave.

- **Prebiotics & Probiotics:** Prebiotics are the fuel your good bacteria love. Think garlic, onions, bananas, and oats. Probiotics are actually live, beneficial bacteria – you'll find them in fermented foods like yogurt, kimchi, and sauerkraut.

- **The "Bad" Stuff? Moderation Is Key:** Sugar, refined carbs, unhealthy fats... these feed the bad gut bacteria and create inflammation. They don't have to be completely off-limits, but they're not the stars of the show.

- **Hydration Matters!** Water keeps everything moving smoothly through your digestive system and helps maintain the delicate balance in your gut.

3. The Gut Cleanse: A Jumpstart, NOT a Cure-All

A 15-day gut cleanse, especially one inspired by O'Neill's focus on natural healing, is a fantastic way to hit the reset button. Think of it as clearing out the gunk, replenishing the good bacteria, and reducing inflammation. But, here's what too many cleanse programs don't tell you:

- **Sustainability is Vital:** If you just go back to eating junk afterward, your gut will too! Think of this cleanse as the beginning of a healthier relationship with food.

- **It's Individual:** Your specific cleanse may involve some temporary dietary changes tailored to your needs.

- **Mindset Matters:** Cleanses can trigger unhealthy food obsession and guilt. Focus on how GOOD you feel when you nourish your body – that's the key to lasting change.

4. Why "Balanced" Beats "Extreme" Every Time

Think of the difference between building a sandcastle and building a fortress. Fad diets are like those flimsy sandcastles – they look impressive for about five seconds, then crumble. A balanced diet, focused on gut health, is your fortress. It takes consistent effort, but here's what you get:

- **Energy That Lasts:** No more sugar crashes or afternoon brain fog.

- **Weight Loss (If That's Your Goal):** But the healthy, sustainable kind.

- **Lifelong Protection:** Strong gut = less likely to develop chronic diseases down the road.

- **You're In Charge:** Not reliant on overpriced supplements or rigid meal plans.

- **You ENJOY Food!:** It's not about punishment! It's about finding healthy things that taste amazing.

The Power of Balance: Not Just What You Eat, But How

Here's the thing: it's not just the food on your plate, it's your whole approach. A balanced diet also includes:

- **Mindful Eating:** Slow down, ditch the distractions, and savor your food. You'll eat less and digest better.

- **Portion Control:** All-you-can-eat buffets aren't doing you any favors. It's about nourishing yourself, not stuffing yourself.

- **Hydration:** Water is life. It helps with digestion, flushes out toxins, and keeps your whole system running smoothly.

- **Regular Movement:** Your body is designed to move! Even a daily walk makes a huge difference to your overall health.

Don't Be Fooled: The Balanced Diet Revolution

I know, "balanced" doesn't sound super exciting, but trust me, it's revolutionary. It's about freedom from:

- **Restrictive Diets:** No more feeling deprived or guilty for enjoying a treat now and then.

- **Food Confusion:** Forget conflicting trends, a balanced diet is timeless and backed by decades of research.

- **Chronic Health Battles:** Take control of your health and feel your best by feeding your body right.

Your Real-Life Guide to Balance (Let's Get Practical!)

Alright, enough talk, let's make this happen. Here's a breakdown of what a balanced diet looks like:

- **Fill Half Your Plate with the Good Stuff:** Load up on fruits, veggies, and whole grains. Aim for a rainbow of colors for maximum nutrients.

- **The Protein Powerhouse:** Include lean meats, fish, beans, lentils, eggs, nuts, and seeds at most meals.

- **Fats, But Choose Wisely:** Stick to olive oil, avocados, nuts, and fatty fish. Limit the saturated and trans fats.

- **Dairy (or the Alternatives):** Aim for lower-fat options, or go for calcium-fortified plant-based milk.

- **Treats in Moderation:** It's okay to have a piece of cake or a glass of wine. It's about the overall 80/20 balance.

Don't try to overhaul everything overnight. Small, sustainable changes add up to big results.

- Start by adding one more serving of fruits or veggies each day.

- Swap sugary drinks for water or herbal tea.

- Cook at home more often so you control what goes into your meals.

This is about feeling amazing, not just looking a certain way. A balanced diet is your key to unlocking boundless energy, good health, and a long, fulfilling life. Isn't that worth giving it a shot?

CHAPTER 5

Benefits of Probiotics and Prebiotics

"The greatest wealth is health." – Virgil

Forget fancy skincare routines and gym memberships, because the real secret to lasting health and vitality lies somewhere a bit less glamorous: your gut. And trust me, what's going on down there impacts a whole lot more than just your bathroom breaks. We're talking about your immune system, your mood, and even how fast those extra pounds seem to cling on.

So, what exactly are these things?

- **Probiotics:** Think of these as the "good guys." Live bacteria and yeasts that naturally live in your body. You find them in fermented foods like yogurt or supplements. Probiotics are like reinforcements for your gut's defense system.

- **Prebiotics:** These are the fuel that keeps those good bacteria thriving. They're a special type of fiber that your body can't digest but your gut bacteria gobble up with glee. You'll find them in stuff like bananas, garlic, onions, and whole grains.

Why Your Gut Microbiome is Running the Show

Your gut is home to tons of microorganisms – it's a whole bustling world in there! This collection of bacteria, fungi, and other friends is your gut microbiome. When everything's in balance, it's a well-oiled machine keeping you healthy. But when the bad guys outnumber the good, then the trouble begins:

- **Weak Immune System:** Like, catching every single cold that goes around, and allergies going haywire. 70% of your immune system lives in your gut, so if it's out of whack, you're a sitting duck.

- **Digestive Nightmares:** We're talking embarrassing gas, bloating, constipation...the gut problems no one wants to discuss openly.

- **Brain Fog and Mood Swings:** Surprise! Your gut produces tons of serotonin, the neurotransmitter that keeps you happy. A messed-up gut messes with your head.

- **Weight Loss Resistance:** Gut bacteria even play a role in how your body uses calories and stores fat. An imbalanced gut can sabotage even your best diet efforts.

- **Serious Long-Term Risks:** Chronic gut imbalance is linked to stuff you don't want – things like heart disease, diabetes, even some cancers.

How do probiotics and prebiotics help?

These little powerhouses work together to bring your gut back to its former glory:

Benefits of Probiotics

- **Boosting good bacteria:** Think back to those friendly bacteria reinforcements. Probiotics deliver a healthy dose, crowding out the troublemakers and restoring order.

- **Better digestion:** They ease those embarrassing gut troubles *and* help you absorb nutrients properly, turning that healthy food into real energy.

- **Immunity Upgrade:** A balanced gut means a stronger immune response. Fewer sick days and less misery, please!

- **Mind Matters:** Better gut health can mean less anxiety, clearer thinking, and a more positive outlook. Who wouldn't want that?

- **Potential Long-Term Protection:** Early research is super promising! Probiotics might even play a role in managing chronic conditions like inflammatory bowel disease or even reducing the risk of certain cancers.

Benefits of Prebiotics

- **Fueling the Good:** Prebiotics are superfoods for your gut's resident good guys, helping them flourish and keep the harmful guys in check.

- **Improved Digestion:** Prebiotics bulk up your stool and promote regularity. They make things move smoothly down there.

- **Calcium Absorption:** Ever noticed prebiotics added to milk? That's because they help your body use the calcium for strong bones.

- **Potential Blood Sugar Control:** Some evidence suggests prebiotics might help manage blood sugar spikes, which is great news for anyone concerned about diabetes.

Science-based benefits of the above claim

- **Conditions Where Probiotics Show Promise:**

  - Diarrhea (especially antibiotic-associated diarrhea)
  - Irritable Bowel Syndrome (IBS)
  - Eczema
  - Ulcerative Colitis
  - Vaginal health
  - Gum disease

- **The Prebiotic Stars:** Look for these fiber types for max gut benefits:

  - Fructooligosaccharides (FOS): Found in onions, garlic, bananas, asparagus, Jerusalem artichokes, and leeks.

  - Galactooligosaccharides (GOS): Naturally occurring in human breast milk, and also added to some food products.

  - Inulin: Present in chicory root, garlic, onions, Jerusalem artichokes, and leeks.

  - Resistant starch: Found in slightly green bananas, cooked and cooled potatoes, rice, and legumes.

  - Beta-glucans: Present in oats, barley, and mushrooms.

  - Pectins: Found in apples, berries, citrus fruits, and carrots.

How Do I Get More Probiotics and Prebiotics?

There are two main ways to get your gut health boost:

1. **Food First:** This is where Hippocrates would be high-fiving you. Load up on these yummy sources:

   - **Probiotic Powerhouses:**

     - Yogurt (look for "live and active cultures")

- Kefir (a tart, drinkable yogurt)
- Sauerkraut (unpasteurized is best)
- Kimchi
- Miso
- Tempeh
- Kombucha (watch the sugar content)

- **Prebiotic All-Stars:**

  - Garlic
  - Onions
  - Leeks
  - Bananas (slightly underripe are better)
  - Oats
  - Apples
  - Flaxseeds
  - Jerusalem artichokes

2. **Supplements: Your Backup Plan**

   - Talk to Your Doctor: Especially if you have any health conditions, it's always a good idea to check with a professional before starting any supplement.

   - Choose Quality: Look for a reputable brand that lists specific strains and CFUs (colony-forming units – basically how many live bacteria you're getting).

   - Refrigerate: Many probiotics need to stay chilled to keep those bacteria alive.

   - Timing Matters: Talk to your doctor or check product directions, as some probiotics work best taken on an empty stomach, others with food.

A Few Things to Keep in Mind

- **"More is Better" Doesn't Apply Here:** Megadosing on either probiotics or prebiotics can backfire, causing gas and bloating. Slow and steady wins the gut health race.

- **Not a Magic Cure-All**: While probiotics and prebiotics offer tons of benefits, they're part of a healthy lifestyle, not a substitute for healthy eating and basic self-care.

- **You Might Notice...Changes:** Increased gas or mild digestive upset in the beginning is common as your gut adjusts. Give it some time, and if the issues are bad, talk to your doctor.

- **Patience is Key:** Don't expect overnight miracles. Gut healing takes time, but sticking with it can pay off BIG TIME in the long run.

So, Where Does That Leave Us?

Your gut is a complex, powerful ecosystem, and probiotics and prebiotics are amazing allies to have in your health journey. They're not a replacement for listening to your body or seeking medical advice when needed. But think of them as a superpower you didn't know you had!

By making gut-friendly choices every day, whether through delicious food or quality supplements, you're investing in a healthier, happier future. Who wouldn't sign up for that?

A final note, as amazing as this all is, understanding your gut microbiome is a constantly evolving area of science. New research is coming out all the time, so stay curious, stay informed, and never stop learning about the incredible power of your body!

CHAPTER 6

Importance of Hydration and Fiber Intake

"A healthy outside starts from the inside." – Robert Urich

Forget miracle serums and fad diets; the real fountain of youth lies in two things you probably overlook daily: water and fiber. See, your body's no fool. It screams for basic nourishment, yet we drown it in sugary sodas, choke it with processed junk, and wonder why we feel like garbage. Listen up, this isn't some preachy health lecture; it's a wake-up call. Ignore your body's needs, and not only will you look and feel your age way too soon, but you're setting yourself up for a whole host of chronic diseases. Let's change that, starting with the dynamic duo of hydration and fiber.

What's the Big Deal with Water?

Yeah, it's everywhere, but are you drinking enough? Your body is not a camel; it can't go days without a decent intake. Here's why H2O is your non-negotiable BFF:

- **Your Body Is Basically a Big Water Balloon:** Around 60% of your body weight is water! Every cell, every organ needs it to function. Get dehydrated, and everything starts malfunctioning.

- **Waste Disposal Service:** Water is how your body flushes out toxins. Not drinking enough? Hello constipation, kidney stones, and a buildup of nasty stuff you don't want lingering.

- **Temperature Control:** Ever sweat? That's your body's natural cooling system, and it relies on water. Get overheated, and it's not just uncomfortable – it can be dangerous.

- **Joint Lubricant:** Achy knees, stiff back? Water keeps your joints happy and helps prevent injuries.

- **It Might Even Help You Lose Weight:** Studies are a bit mixed, but some suggest drinking water before meals can help with feeling full and reduce your overall calorie intake.

How Much Water is Enough?

There's no single magic number for everyone, but here's the gist:

- **The General Rule:** You've heard "8 glasses a day," but that's oversimplified. Aim for half your body weight in ounces. So, weigh 150 pounds? Shoot for 75 ounces of water daily.

- **Listen to Your Thirst...Mostly:** Feeling parched is your body's signal for more. But don't wait until then, keep sipping throughout the day.

- **Check Your Pee:** Sorry, but yeah. It should be pale yellow, not dark. Dark pee means you're dehydrated.

What About Fiber?

It's so much more than just keeping you regular (although that's important too!). Fiber is the indigestible part of plant foods, and it's highly beneficial:

- **Two Types, Both Matter:**

  - **Soluble Fiber:** Dissolves in water, turning into a gel-like substance in your gut. This slows digestion, helps you feel full, and is amazing for cholesterol control. Find it in oats, beans, apples, and citrus fruits.

  - **Insoluble Fiber:** The poop specialist! This type doesn't dissolve, adding bulk to your stool and making things move along smoothly. Think whole grains, leafy greens, and the skins of fruits and veggies.

- **Gut Bacteria's Favorite Meal:** This is where fiber gets really cool! Those trillions of gut microbes we talked about? They feast on fiber. A well-fed gut microbiome = a happy, healthy body.

- **Heart Health Booster:** Soluble fiber, specifically, can help lower LDL cholesterol, reducing your risk of heart disease.

- **Blood Sugar Management:** Fiber slows the absorption of sugar, preventing those nasty spikes that leave you feeling hungry and reaching for junk.

- **Weight Management:** Feeling full and satisfied thanks to fiber means less temptation to overeat. Plus, a healthy gut supports a healthy metabolism.

Scientific benefits of hydration and fiber

We've got mountains of research on the benefits of hydration and fiber:

- **The Energy Boost:** Even mild dehydration can decrease alertness and cognitive performance in both men and women. (See: *Van Nieuwenhoven et al., 2001*)

- **The Kidney Stone Blocker:** One study suggests increasing fluid intake decreases recurrence risk in kidney stone patients by about 60%. BAM! (Borghi et al., 1996)

- **The Poop Problem Solver:** Increasing fiber intake significantly improves stool frequency and consistency for those dealing with constipation. (Yang et al., 2012)

- **The Blood Sugar Stabilizer:** Fiber-rich diets lead to better blood sugar control and reduced insulin spikes. Good news, especially for those at risk for type 2 diabetes (Chandalia et al., 2000)

- **Dehydration Dangers:** Even mild dehydration impairs concentration, mood, and physical performance. Long-term, it increases your risk of chronic conditions like kidney disease and even some cancers.

- **Fiber and Disease Prevention:** Studies strongly link high-fiber diets to reduced risk of heart disease, stroke, type 2 diabetes, and colorectal cancer. We're talking major protection!

- **The Mind-Gut Connection:** Your gut bacteria fueled by fiber play a role in everything from your immune system to your mood. This area is still being explored, but the potential benefits are huge.

CHAPTER 7

Managing Stress and Sleep for Gut Health

"The greatest weapon against stress is our ability to choose one thought over another."
– William James

They say "You are what you eat," but the truth is, you're also how you sleep...and how much your brain is freaking out. Stress and lack of sleep are gut health saboteurs, plain and simple. Remember how the food industry and Big Pharma don't want you thriving? Well, guess what? Chronic stress and sleepless nights are their evil allies. Here's the deal: what happens in your head directly messes with your gut, kickstarting a whole chain reaction of health problems you wouldn't even think to connect. In previous chapters, we have spoken a bit about stress and how it negatively affects our guts, let's continue to expose the truth about the subject matter and arm ourselves with the tools to take control.

The Vicious Cycle: How Stress Hacks Your Gut

1. **Fight or Flight Gone Wild:** Our bodies have this ancient survival mechanism. The brain dumps stress hormones (cortisol is the main culprit), digestion shuts down, and we run like hell. The problem is, modern stress – traffic jams, work deadlines, relationship drama – triggers that same reaction, but we're just sitting there stewing in the toxic stress bath.

2. **Leaky Gut Incoming:** Your gut lining is supposed to be a tightly-knit barrier, letting good stuff in, and keeping bad stuff out. Chronic stress punches holes in that barrier, leading to a "leaky gut." Now toxins, undigested food, and all sorts of nasty things leak into your bloodstream where they don't belong.

3. **Microbiome Mayhem:** Your friendly gut bacteria take a serious hit from stress. The balance gets thrown off, paving the way for harmful bacteria to take over. This messes with digestion, immunity... your entire body's command center.

4. **Welcome to Inflammation City:** Leaky gut and messed-up gut bacteria equal one thing: **INFLAMMATION**. This is the root of so many problems: achy joints, weight loss resistance, and even depression. Your gut is literally on fire.

And That's Not All...Stress Also Leads to:

- **Crappy Food Choices:** Does anyone else reach for cookies instead of carrots when stressed? Stress fries your decision-making centers and makes junk food seem irresistible.

- **Digestive Distress:** Constipation, diarrhea, bloating – stress can make your bathroom routine a total nightmare.

- **Zero Motivation to Exercise:** This is a bummer because exercise is a great stress-buster and helps your gut!

Sleep Deprivation: The Gut's Worst Enemy

Think pulling all-nighters and barely scraping 5 hours is no big deal? Your gut strongly disagrees.

- **Microbiome Madness:** Just a few nights of bad sleep disrupts your gut bacteria just like chronic stress does. You're basically setting yourself up for all those problems we just talked about.

- **Ghrelin the Hunger Monster:** Sleep deprivation spikes "ghrelin," the hormone that makes you ravenous. At the same time, it lowers "leptin" which tells you you're full. Recipe for overeating, especially junk cravings.

- **Inflammation Strikes Again:** Not getting enough sleep sends those inflammatory signals through the roof, adding fuel to the gut health fire.

What Can You Do About It?

We are not going to lie, modern life makes consistent Zen and 8-hour nights a real challenge. But that doesn't mean your gut has to suffer eternally! Here's the battle plan:

Stress Management Toolkit

- **Movement is Medicine:** This is non-negotiable. Exercise doesn't have to be a marathon...a brisk walk, dancing in your kitchen, anything that gets you moving and releases some of those stress hormones.

- **Mindfulness Matters:** Meditation, deep breathing...sounds cliché, but it works. Even 5 minutes a day trains your brain to handle stress without freaking out. There are tons of apps if you need guidance.

- **Nature Therapy:** Sunshine, fresh air, listening to birds...it's amazing how getting outside resets your nervous system.

- **Connection is Key:** Spend time with people who make you laugh, and who support you. Feeling isolated makes stress so much worse.

- **Sleep Hygiene 101:** This is a whole topic on its own, but the basics: dark, cool room, no screens before bed, and stick to a regular sleep schedule as much as possible.

- **Adaptogenic Herbs:** Things like Ashwagandha and Holy Basil have some science backing them for stress relief. Always talk to your doctor first, especially if you take other medications.

Gut-Soothing Nutrition

- **Whole Foods FTW:** Processed junk = gut misery. Focus on real, unprocessed foods as much as possible: veggies, fruits, whole grains, lean protein.

- **Fermented Friends:** Load up on those probiotic powerhouses (yogurt, kimchi, etc.) to rebuild your gut army.

- **Prebiotic Power:** Garlic, onions, bananas...feed those good bacteria so they can thrive.

- **Manage Caffeine and Alcohol:** Both disrupt sleep AND irritate your gut. Notice how they affect you and scale back if needed.

- **Hydration Station:** Water keeps things moving smoothly and helps your whole body function better.

Jude's Experience

I am Jude and it's a pleasure to meet you. For the past 7 years, my body has felt like a stranger to me. I used to be the guy who could eat anything, stay out late, and still feel energized the next day. But 3 years ago, it became a struggle. The bloating, the fatigue, the constant trips to the bathroom - it felt like my body was revolting against me.

I tried all the quick fixes – trendy diets, cutting out carbs, even those weird "cleansing" teas that promised miracles. Nothing made a lasting difference. I was getting desperate. Then a friend shared something about a link of Barbara O'Neill's natural remedies which contained natural ways for living a better and healthier life. Resources about her filled the internet after she was banned for life from providing any health services in Australia in 2019. This action made Barbara more popular and many of my friends adopted her teachings and are still living testimonies to their optimal health.

Now back to my experience... Honestly, I was skeptical but figured I had nothing to lose.

The first few days surprised me. It wasn't about deprivation but about *adding* whole foods, prebiotics, and probiotics. It was like finally giving my body the good stuff it craved. Suddenly, I wasn't starving all the time or reaching for energy drinks just to function.

I was starting to feel lighter and energized, especially when I completed the 15-Day Gut Cleanse – courtesy of her teachings. But the real change went deeper than that. All those years of processed food and ignoring my stress had taken a toll. This cleanse felt like I was taking control of my health again.

It wasn't always easy. There were days when the pizza cravings were intense or times when stress threatened to derail me. But I leaned into the online support group Barbara O'Neill recommended, and they were lifesavers. They shared recipes, tips for managing stress, and reminders that I wasn't alone.

By the end of those 15 days, something shifted. It wasn't just about the bloating getting better, but about feeling more connected to my body. I felt like a new person, I loved my body again, and I was always energetic all through the day. I started moving more, not as some grueling workout, but just taking walks, rediscovering the joy of being active. I started paying attention to how *food* made me feel, not just how it tasted.

The weight loss came gradually but surely. More importantly, I felt strong, clear-headed, and like I could handle whatever life threw my way.

This didn't change my life overnight. It wasn't magic, but it started a process. It inspired me to ditch the old habits that weren't serving me. It wasn't a "diet" so much as a reset - a way to finally start listening to my gut.

If you're feeling like I did – tired, frustrated, trapped in a body that doesn't feel like yours – maybe it's time for your own gut cleanse journey. It will unlock a healthier, happier you. I know it was for me.

PART 3: 15-DAY GUT CLEANSE TO A NEW YOU

CHAPTER 8

Take advantage of the Gut C.A.R.E Program to eliminate symptoms and maintain a healthy Gut

"The health of your gut is the key to your overall health. When your gut is happy, you feel better from head to toe." – Dr. Josh Axe

Aside from the effective nature of the 15-Day Gut Cleanse which we will discuss shortly, another powerful Gut Cleansing tool is the ***Gut C.A.R.E Program***. It was birthed by Dr. Vincent Pedre using his experience from IBS for several years. This led him to become an expert in functional medicine and learning how to heal his body from within.

Remember how you feel on your best days – energized, clear-headed, and just overall well? That's often a direct reflection of a happy, healthy gut. But what about those other days when things feel "off"? Bloating, gas, indigestion, mood swings, brain fog... your gut might be trying to tell you it needs some extra TLC.

The Gut C.A.R.E. Program isn't just about a 15-day cleanse. It's a framework designed to help you understand your gut, heal it, and give it the long-term support it needs to keep you feeling your best. Let's break down what C.A.R.E. stands for and how each step plays a role in your journey to optimal gut health.

Why We Need to C.A.R.E

I get it, maybe you're thinking, "Well, this all sounds great, but why bother? Is this going to be worth it?" Absolutely! Think back to those nagging, everyday symptoms that never seem to go away – the bloating, the fatigue, the cravings, the mood swings. These aren't just annoying; they're signs that your gut has been trying to tell you something's wrong for a while. The gut is often called our "second brain." Its health is intricately tied to our overall health – physically and mentally.

When we follow the C.A.R.E. Program, we're hitting the reset button. We're giving our gut the chance to recover, helping it get back to its main job – digesting food, absorbing nutrients, and protecting us from all sorts of health issues.

Breaking Down the Gut C.A.R.E. Program

Alright, let's dive into each step one by one!

Step 1 - CLEANSE

In the "Cleanse" stage, the name of the game is elimination. We're removing three key sources of trouble:

1. **Food sensitivities:** Common culprits like gluten, dairy, soy, corn, and others can wreak havoc, even if you don't have full-blown allergies. We'll cut them out for a while to let your gut calm down.

2. **Inflammatory substances:** Think sugar, processed foods, refined carbs, and not-so-great fats. These all promote inflammation, making it harder for your gut to heal. We're replacing them with a focus on whole, natural foods.

3. **Gut irritants:** We're ditching things like coffee and alcohol which upset healthy gut function. And we're getting extra-careful about how we prepare our food (cleaning up that kitchen, remember?!) to avoid environmental toxins that mess up our gut bacteria balance.

The "Cleanse" step isn't meant to starve you! You'll be eating plenty of delicious, nourishing food based on a simple shopping list. We're just removing the junk to give your gut a break!

Step 2 - ACTIVATE

Think of digestion as a well-oiled machine with different parts working together. Your stomach produces acid, your pancreas and gallbladder send in enzymes, and so on. When your gut is out of balance, all these parts can get stressed and out of sync. The "Activate" stage is about giving them support!

Digestive enzyme supplements help break down your food, taking some of the pressure off your system. This is super-important because undigested food particles can actually cause more inflammation! Plus, if you've got low stomach acid, we might add a supplement to support that.

Step 3 – RESTORE

This is where the magic of friendly bacteria (also called probiotics) comes in! Our guts are supposed to be filled with a thriving community of these little guys. They help keep everything working smoothly with these cool benefits:

- **Fighting off the bad guys:** Probiotics make it harder for harmful bacteria, yeast, and parasites to take hold.

- **Supporting our immune system:** A lot of our immune function is actually centered in the gut!

- **Boosting our mood:** Believe it or not, our gut bacteria can even influence how we feel mentally.

So, in the "Restore" stage, we replenish those beneficial bugs. We do this through a high-quality probiotic supplement and fermented foods that support a diverse and healthy gut microbiome.

Step 4 – ENHANCE

In this final stage, we focus on healing the actual lining of your gut. Imagine your digestive tract is lined with a protective barrier. When it's healthy, it does its job of keeping out things that don't belong. But inflammation can damage it, leading to something called "leaky gut". That means little bits of food, toxins, and microbes can leak into your bloodstream, wreaking havoc!

This is when supplements like L-glutamine, DGL, aloe vera, omega-3, and zinc step in. They work to soothe and repair that lining, kind of like applying a bandaid and super-charged ointment to a wound. This helps restore your gut's natural defenses and prevent even more inflammation!

Your Gut C.A.R.E Journey: What to Expect

The Gut C.A.R.E. Program comes **with a handy template and supplement recommendations**. It's a day-by-day guide helping you put the steps into practice. You'll see when to take which supplements, meal ideas, and even some tips for managing those initial detox symptoms!

Here's a peek at what a typical day might look like:

- **Morning:** Start with lemon water, a gratitude practice, and maybe some gentle yoga. Then, it's time for a nutrient-packed breakfast smoothie packed with gut-friendly ingredients. You'll take your first round of supplements around this time.

- **Lunch and Dinner:** Focus on meals built from the Happy Gut Diet shopping list – proteins, healthy fats, and tons of veggies. Don't forget those digestive enzymes!

- **Throughout the Day:** Aim for plenty of clean water and keep an eye on your symptom journal. You might try some additional snacks as needed (sticking to gut-healthy options, of course).

- **Evening Routine:** Before bed, take your last round of supplements. A little calming meditation will help prepare you for a restful night's sleep.

Here's a realistic look at what you might experience as your body adjusts:

- **The First Few Days:** This is when you might feel some detox symptoms. Headaches, and a little fatigue – this is a sign that your body is cleaning house! Don't worry, it'll pass with plenty of water and rest.

- **The First Week:** As you eliminate the bad and boost the good, you might notice improvements already! Less bloating, more energy, better focus – even your mood might start to lift a bit.

- **The Second Week:** This is where things start to solidify. Your cravings will diminish, and you'll feel more satisfied with smaller portions of healthy food. Digestion improves, and those stubborn ailments begin fading away.

- **Beyond Two Weeks:** Congrats! You've completed the core program. Now, it's about maintaining those healthy habits. You'll find reintroducing some "treat" foods will be easier, but you'll likely notice that they don't make you feel as great as before.

The Power of a Happy Gut

The Gut C.A.R.E. Program isn't just about temporary fixes. It's about creating long-lasting habits that make you feel your best. Here's what you can expect with a happy and healthy gut:

- **Boosted Energy:** Finally, you won't feel tired mid-afternoon! With proper digestion, your body receives steady energy from the food you eat.

- **Weight Management:** When your gut is in balance, cravings subside, and your metabolism works efficiently. Losing any extra weight or maintaining a healthy weight becomes so much easier.

- **Clarity and Focus:** That "brain fog" is your gut trying to tell you something! You'll be amazed at how much better you can think when gut inflammation is reduced.

- **Improved Mood:** Your gut produces many of the chemicals that affect your mood. A healthy gut often translates to less anxiety and a more positive outlook.

- **Stronger Immunity:** Your gut is a huge part of your immune system. With it in tip-top shape, you'll get sick less often and bounce back quicker.

Maintaining Your Results after the Gut C.A.R.E Program

The Gut C.A.R.E Program isn't a quicky. It's about creating sustainable changes. The good news is, that once the initial 28 days are up, you'll be equipped with knowledge to keep your gut happy for the long haul! Here's how:

- **Food Reintroduction:** You'll slowly reintroduce certain foods to see how they affect you now that your gut is healed. This lets you personalize your diet in a way that works for your body!

- **Supplements:** You may still benefit from some of the supplements, especially probiotics and enzymes. Work with a healthcare practitioner to figure out what's best for your individual needs.

- **Mindset:** Remember those gratitude practices and moments of mindful eating we talked about? Keep them going! Stress is a major gut disruptor, so finding ways to manage it is key.

- **Listen to your body:** It's your best guide to long-term gut health. Pay attention to how different foods, situations, or even medications might make you feel.

Making the C.A.R.E. Program Your Lifestyle

Here are some tips to make these changes last:

- **Be Patient and Kind to Yourself:** Nobody's Perfect. If you slip up, don't give up! Just get back on track with your next meal.

- **Listen to Your Body:** Pay attention to how different foods make you feel. That's the best guide for what works for you.

- **Mindfulness and Stress Management:** Stress takes a toll on your gut. Find ways to relax – it might be yoga, a walk in nature, or just a few deep breaths.

- **Stay Connected:** Find support from a friend, or family member, or find an online community that understands your journey.

Friend, you have the power to transform how you feel! The Gut C.A.R.E. Program is your roadmap to a healthier, happier you. I believe in you! When you commit to caring for your gut, you're giving yourself the greatest gift. And with all the amazing benefits, why wait? Start your gut-healing journey today!

Remember:

- Your gut is unique, so some adjustments might be needed. If you have pre-existing health conditions, always consult your doctor before starting any new program.

- Consider finding a functional medicine practitioner who can provide additional support and personalization for your gut health journey.

The choice to take control of your gut health is a powerful one. I believe in you! The Gut C.A.R.E. Program is designed to give you the tools and knowledge you need to succeed. Let's get started on this journey as we unveil the 15-Day Gut Cleanse to better health – you deserve to feel your best!

CHAPTER 9

15-Day Gut Cleanse Plan

Here's a comprehensive 15-Day Gut Cleanse Plan, presented in tabular form and incorporating the concepts of Reinforce, Cleanse, and Replenish. I've also integrated scientific support for the dietary strategies involved.

Important Considerations:

- **Adaptability:** This is a sample plan; adjust it based on your dietary needs and preferences.

- **Consultation:** It's wise to consult a healthcare professional before starting any cleanse, especially if you have underlying health conditions.

- **Hydration:** Drink plenty of water throughout the cleanse to aid digestion and toxin removal.

- **Mindfulness:** Pay attention to how your body feels and adjust as needed.

The 15-Day Gut Cleanse

- **Stage 1: Reinforce (Days 1-5)** Focus on nourishing your gut with prebiotic-rich foods to support existing beneficial bacteria.

- **Stage 2: Cleanse (Days 6-10):** Gently stimulate detoxification pathways with fiber, hydrating fluids, and targeted herbs or supplements (consult your healthcare provider).

- **Stage 3: Replenish (Days 11-15)** Focus on probiotic-rich foods and easy-to-digest options to repopulate healthy gut bacteria and promote overall gut health.

Dietary Guidelines

- **Emphasis:** Whole, unprocessed foods, fruits, vegetables, healthy fats, lean proteins, complex carbs.

- **Minimize:** Processed foods, refined sugars, excessive red meat, artificial sweeteners, and inflammatory oils.

- **Possible Supplements:** Discuss with your doctor options like gentle fiber supplements, magnesium citrate (for regularity), digestive enzymes, or a targeted probiotic.

15-Day Gut Cleanse Plan in a table

Day	Stage	Breakfast	Lunch	Dinner	Notes
Day 1	Reinforce	Oatmeal with berries, nuts, seeds	Veggie and lentil soup	Salmon with roasted vegetables	Focus on fiber
Day 2	Reinforce	Fermented yogurt (unsweetened) with fruit	Big salad with grilled chicken or tofu	Lentil stew with brown rice	Include fermented foods
Day 3	Reinforce	Eggs with avocado and whole-grain toast	Leftovers from lentil stew	Roasted chicken with sweet potato and greens	
Day 4	Reinforce	Smoothie with greens, protein powder, berries	Quinoa salad with chickpeas and veggies	Salmon with steamed broccoli	Stay hydrated
Day 5	Reinforce	Chia pudding with fruit	Chicken or veggie wrap with whole-wheat tortilla	Tuna salad with mixed greens	Consider a gentle herbal tea
Day 6	Cleanse	Green juice (cucumber, celery, spinach, etc.)	Salad with lean protein and mixed greens	Light vegetable soup with broth	Up water intake. Consider adding a fiber supplement (discuss with your doctor)
Day 7	Cleanse	Smoothie with greens, fruit, and protein	Big salad with light dressing, add beans/lentils	Clear broth with veggies or bone broth	

Day 8	Cleanse	Warm lemon water	Vegetable soup with quinoa or rice	Steamed fish and vegetables	Consider magnesium citrate for gentle bowel support (discuss with your doctor)
Day 9	Cleanse	Smoothie with plant-based protein and fruit	Salad with legumes for protein	Kitchari (Ayurvedic lentil and rice stew)	
Day 10	Cleanse	Overnight oats with berries	Lentil soup	Vegetable stir-fry with tofu or tempeh	
Day 11	Replenish	Fermented yogurt with fruit and nuts	Salad with grilled fish or tofu	Chicken vegetable soup	Probiotic focus
Day 12	Replenish	Eggs with whole-grain toast and avocado	Salad with quinoa and roasted veggies	Baked fish with sweet potato	
Day 13	Replenish	Smoothie with greens, berries, yogurt	Big salad with mixed greens and protein	Lentil stew	Continue fermented foods
Day 14	Replenish	Oatmeal with fruit and seeds	Leftovers from lentil stew	Veggie burger with sweet potato fries	
Day 15	Replenish	Chia pudding with fruit and nuts	Salad with lean protein	Salmon and roasted vegetables	

Remember, listen to your body and adjust portions or meals as needed. This cleanse is intended as a supportive tool for long-term gut health!

A Healthy Gut's Grocery List

Acceptable Foods (Promote Gut Health)

- **Fruits**

  1. **Berries:** Blueberries, raspberries, strawberries, blackberries (rich in antioxidants and fiber)

  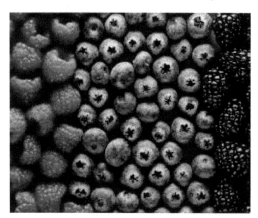

  2. **Apples:** Good source of pectin, a type of soluble fiber

  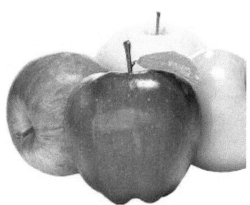

  3. **Bananas:** Contain prebiotics and potassium

  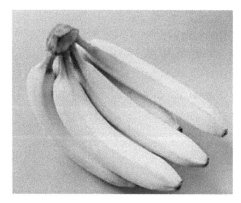

  4. **Citrus fruits:** Oranges, grapefruits, lemons (vitamin C and fiber)

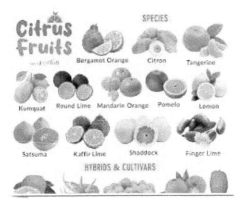

5. **Avocados:** Healthy fats and fiber

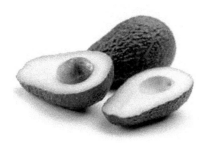

- **Vegetables**

6. **Cruciferous vegetables:** Broccoli, cauliflower, Brussels sprouts (prebiotic-rich)

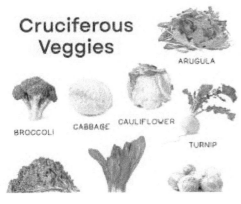

7. **Leafy Greens:** Spinach, kale, Swiss chard (vitamins, minerals, fiber)

8. **Garlic and Onions:** Contain prebiotic compounds

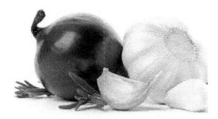

9. **Sweet Potatoes:** Loaded with fiber and antioxidants

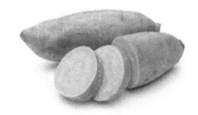

10. **Asparagus:** Excellent prebiotic source

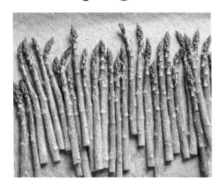

- **Whole Grains**

11. **Oats:** High in soluble fiber (beta-glucans)

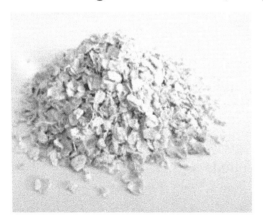

12. Quinoa: Complete protein, a good source of fiber

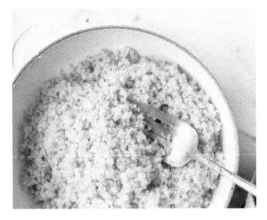

13. Brown Rice: Fiber-rich, magnesium

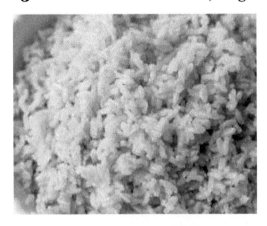

14. Whole-wheat bread: More fiber than white bread

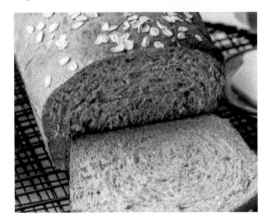

- **Legumes**

15. **Lentils:** Protein, fiber, and prebiotics

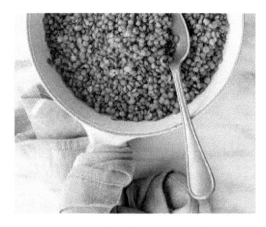

16. **Beans (kidney, black, pinto):** Excellent source of fiber

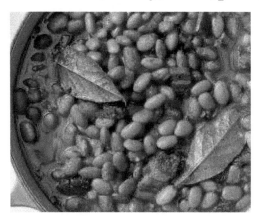

17. **Chickpeas:** Versatile and fiber-packed

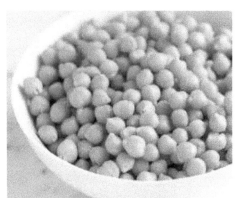

- **Fermented Foods**

18. **Yogurt (with live cultures):** Probiotics for gut health

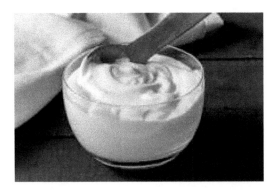

19.**Kefir:** Fermented milk drink, rich in probiotics

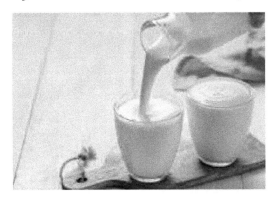

20. **Sauerkraut:** Fermented cabbage, beneficial bacteria

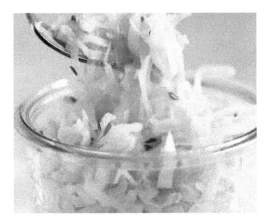

21.**Kimchi:** Spicy Korean fermented vegetables

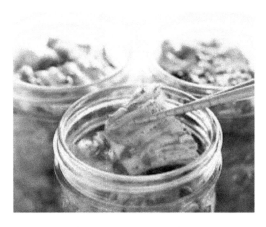

22.   **Miso:** Fermented soybean paste, probiotics

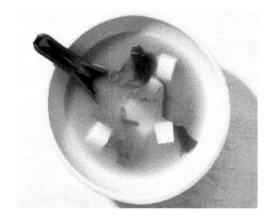

- **Healthy Fats**

23. **Nuts (almonds, walnuts):** Healthy fats, fiber, protein

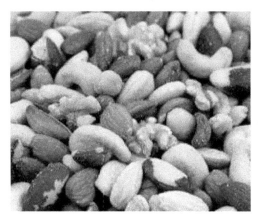

24. **Seeds (chia, flax, pumpkin):** Fiber, omega-3s, protein

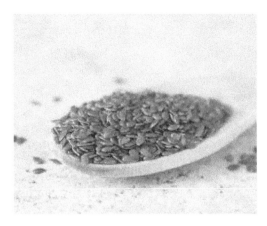

25. **Olive oil:** Anti-inflammatory properties

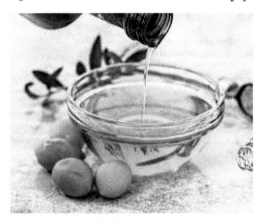

- **Lean Proteins**

26. **Fish (salmon, tuna):** Omega-3 fatty acids for gut health

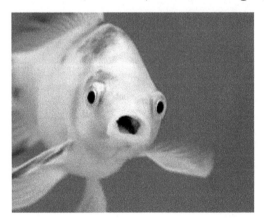

27. **Chicken and turkey (skinless):** Easy to digest

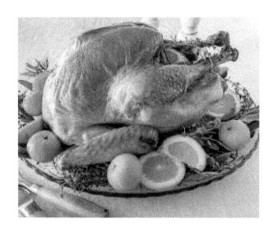

Unacceptable Foods (Can Harm Gut Health)

- **Processed Foods** (Often high in sugar, unhealthy fats, and additives)

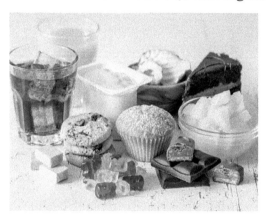

- **Sugary Drinks:** Soda, sweetened juices, sports drinks

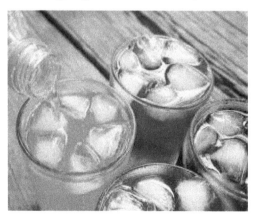

- **Refined Grains:** White bread, white rice, white pasta

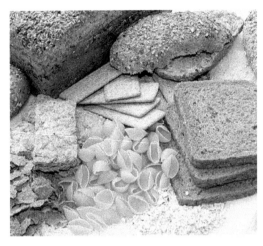

- **Fried Foods:** French fries, fried chicken, etc.

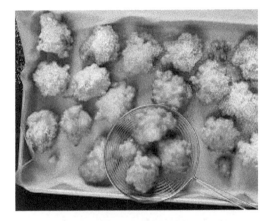

- **Artificial Sweeteners:** Can disrupt gut bacteria balance

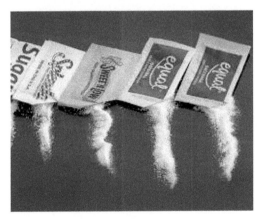

- **Processed Meats:** Bacon, sausage, hot dogs

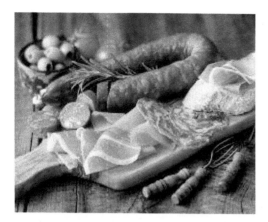

- **Excessive Red Meat:** May increase the risk of gut-related health issues

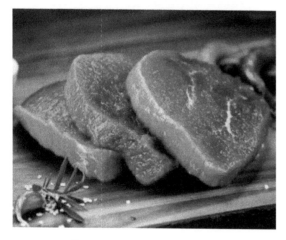

- **Foods High in Saturated and Trans Fats:** Many baked goods, processed snacks

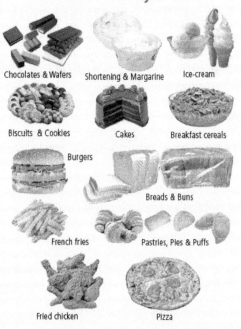

TRANS FAT
is found in many foods

Chocolates & Wafers   Shortening & Margarine   Ice-cream

Biscuits & Cookies   Cakes   Breakfast cereals

Burgers

Breads & Buns

French fries   Pastries, Pies & Puffs

Fried chicken   Pizza

- **Added Sugars:** Candy, cookies, cakes, sugary cereals

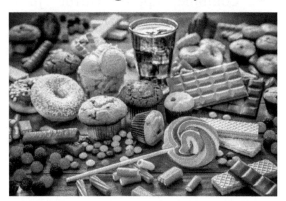

- **Excessive Alcohol:** Disrupts the gut microbiome

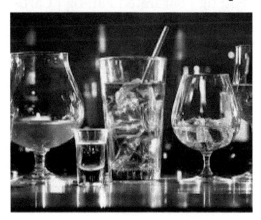

101 HAPPY GUT RECIPES

1. Avocado Orange Smoothie

Preparation Time: 5 Minutes | Total Time: 7 Minutes | Serves: 2

Ingredients:

- 1 cup light almond milk or Homemade Almond Milk
- 2 ounces tempeh
- 1 orange, peeled and seeded
- ½ avocado, pitted and peeled
- ½ cup packed baby spinach
- 1 teaspoon agave nectar

Directions:

1. Place all ingredients into a high-speed blender. If using a traditional blender, consider chopping the orange and tempeh for a smoother blend.

2. Blend until creamy and smooth, ensuring a homogenous texture.

3. Pour into two glasses and enjoy immediately for a fresh, nutrient-rich start to your day.

Nutrition per serving: Calories: 210 | Total Fat: 9g | Saturated Fat: 2g | Carbs: 26g | Fiber: 5g | Protein: 9g | Sodium: 75mg | Vitamin A: 25% DV | Vitamin C: 70% DV

2. Carrot Kombucha Smoothie

Preparation Time: 5 Minutes | Total Time: 7 Minutes | Serves: 2

Ingredients:

- ½ apple, peeled and cored
- ½ cup 100 percent carrot juice
- 3 fresh strawberries, hulled
- 2 ice cubes
- 1 cup Ginger Kombucha or GT's Enlightened Organic Raw Gingerade Kombucha

Directions:

1. Combine apple, carrot juice, strawberries, and ice cubes in a blender, blending until smooth.

2. Pour the mixture into two glasses, then stir in ½ cup of kombucha into each glass.

3. Enjoy immediately or refrigerate and savor within 3 to 4 days, stirring well before serving.

Nutrition per serving: Calories: 60 | Total Fat: 0g | Saturated Fat: 0g | Carbs: 14g | Fiber: 2g | Protein: <1g | Sodium: 50mg | Vitamin A: 180% DV | Vitamin C: 30% DV

3. Carrot Immune Boost

Preparation Time: 5 Minutes | Total Time: 7 Minutes | Serves: 1

Ingredients:

- ½ apple, peeled and cored
- ½ cup 100 percent carrot juice
- ½ cup low-fat or nonfat vanilla bean yogurt
- 3 fresh strawberries, hulled
- 2 ice cubes

Directions:

1. In a blender, mix the apple, carrot juice, yogurt, strawberries, and ice cubes until smooth and creamy.

2. Serve this nutritious concoction immediately, or refrigerate to enjoy later, ensuring you stir well before drinking.

Nutrition per serving: Calories: 220 | Total Fat: 2.5g | Saturated Fat: 1.5g | Carbs: 41g | Fiber: 4g | Protein: 10g | Sodium: 140mg | Vitamin A: 360% DV | Vitamin C: 100% DV

4. Kiwi Strawberry Smoothie

Preparation Time: 5 Minutes | Total Time: 7 Minutes | Serves: 2

Ingredients:

- ½ cup low-fat or nonfat plain Greek yogurt
- ½ cup light almond milk or Homemade Almond Milk

- 2 fresh kiwis, peeled
- 4 to 5 fresh strawberries, hulled
- ¼ avocado, pitted and peeled
- 2 teaspoons honey (optional)

Directions:

1. Combine yogurt, almond milk, kiwis, strawberries, avocado, and honey in a blender and blend until smooth.

2. Divide the smoothie between two glasses for a vibrant, nutrient-packed drink that's perfect for boosting your immune system.

Nutrition per serving: Calories: 170 | Total Fat: 4.5g | Saturated Fat: 0g | Carbs: 26g | Fiber: 5g | Protein: 8g | Sodium: 75mg | Vitamin A: 4% DV | Vitamin C: 180% DV

5. Mango Banana Smoothie

Preparation Time: 5 Minutes | Total Time: 7 Minutes | Serves: 2

Ingredients:

- 1 banana
- 1 cup frozen cubed mango
- ½ cup low-fat or nonfat milk
- ½ cup Vanilla Bean Smoothie or vanilla bean yogurt

Directions:

1. Blend banana, mango, milk, and yogurt until smooth and icy.

2. Pour into glasses and enjoy a tropical escape in every sip,

perfect for a healthy, refreshing treat.

Nutrition per serving: Calories: 160 | Total Fat: 1g | Saturated Fat: 0.5g | Carbs: 34g | Fiber: 3g | Protein: 6g | Sodium: 50mg | Vitamin A: 15% DV | Vitamin C: 45% DV

6. Orange Kombucha

Preparation Time: 6-12 Hours (Infusion Time) | Total Time: Up to 12 Hours and 7 Minutes | Serves: 1

Ingredients:

- 1 cup Original Kombucha or GT's Enlightened Organic Raw Original Kombucha

- 1 orange, cut into 5 or 6 slices

Directions:

1. In a glass jar, combine kombucha with orange slices. Cover tightly and allow the mixture to infuse at room temperature for 6 to 12 hours, depending on your flavor preference.

2. Once infused to your liking, refrigerate to chill. Serve over ice, garnished with fresh orange slices for a refreshing, tangy treat.

Nutrition per serving: Calories: 60 | Total Fat: 0g | Saturated Fat: 0g | Carbs: 13g | Fiber: 2g | Protein: <1g | Sodium: 10mg | Vitamin A: 2% DV | Vitamin C: 45% DV

7. Orange Strawberry Freeze

Preparation Time: 5 Minutes | Total Time: 7 Minutes | Serves: 2

Ingredients:

- 1 cup low-fat or nonfat plain Greek yogurt

- 1 cup frozen strawberries

- ½ cup 100 percent orange juice

- ½ orange, peeled and seeded

- 1 tablespoon honey

- 4 or 5 ice cubes

Directions:

1. Combine yogurt, strawberries, and orange juice in a blender until smooth. Add the orange, honey, and ice cubes, blending until achieving a frosty smoothie texture.

2. Divide the smoothie between two glasses for a refreshing drink that's bursting with vitamin C and flavor.

Nutrition per serving: Calories: 170 | Total Fat: 0g | Saturated Fat: 0g | Carbs: 31g | Fiber: 3g | Protein: 13g | Sodium: 55mg | Vitamin A: 2% DV | Vitamin C: 180% DV

8. Roasted Red Pepper Juice

Preparation Time: 5 Minutes | Total Time: 7 Minutes | Serves: 2

Ingredients:

- 1 cup Orange Power Smoothie

- 1 cup jarred roasted red peppers, drained

- 1 teaspoon organic mellow white miso

- ¼ teaspoon garlic powder

Directions:

1. Combine the Orange Power Smoothie base with roasted red peppers, miso, and garlic powder in a blender, blending until smooth.

2. Serve this unique and savory juice in glasses, offering a potent mix of vitamins A and C for an exceptional immune boost.

Nutrition per serving: Calories: 220 | Total Fat: 2g | Saturated Fat: 0g | Carbs: 58g | Fiber: 5g | Protein: 3g | Sodium: 425mg | Vitamin A: 230% DV | Vitamin C: 450% DV

9. Tangerine Freeze

Preparation Time: 5 Minutes | Total Time: 7 Minutes | Serves: 2

Ingredients:

- 2 fresh tangerines, peeled and seeded

- ½ cup plain kefir or Traditional Plain Kefir

- ½ cup coconut milk beverage

- 1 teaspoon coconut palm sugar (optional)

- 4 or 5 ice cubes

Directions:

1. Combine tangerines, kefir, coconut milk, coconut palm sugar (if desired), and ice cubes in a blender until smooth and frothy.

2. Pour into glasses for a unique and tropical smoothie experience,

blending the sweet flavors of tangerine with the creaminess of kefir and a hint of coconut.

Nutrition per serving: Calories: 120 | Total Fat: 1g | Saturated Fat: 0.5g | Carbs: 25g | Fiber: 3g | Protein: 5g | Sodium: 45mg | Vitamin A: 25% DV | Vitamin C: 70% DV

10. Mango Coconut Kefir

Preparation Time: 5 Minutes | Total Time: 7 Minutes | Serves: 1

Ingredients:

- 1 cup Pineapple Chia Colada Kefir

- 1 cup frozen cubed mango

- 1 tablespoon shredded coconut

Directions:

1. Blend the Pineapple Chia Colada Kefir, mango, and shredded coconut until smooth for a tropical, creamy delight.

2. Pour into a glass and enjoy a rich, flavorful smoothie that's not only delicious but also packed with probiotics and vitamins for your health.

Nutrition per serving: Calories: 250 | Total Fat: 8g | Saturated Fat: 5g | Carbs: 44g | Fiber: 6g | Protein: 5g | Sodium: 50mg | Vitamin A: 30% DV | Vitamin C: 120% DV

11. Arctic Ginger Blue

Preparation Time: 5 Minutes | Total Time: 7 Minutes | Serves: 1

Ingredients:

- 1 cup frozen blueberries
- ½ cup Ginger Beer or store-bought ginger beer
- 1 cup plain seltzer

Directions:

1. Combine the blueberries and Ginger Beer in a blender and blend until smooth.
2. Pour the blueberry-ginger mixture into a glass, top with the seltzer, and stir gently to combine for a refreshing and zesty drink.
3. Enjoy immediately for a burst of flavor and a kick of ginger's anti-inflammatory benefits, complemented by the antioxidants of blueberries.

Nutrition per serving: Calories: 130 | Total Fat: 0g | Saturated Fat: 0g | Carbs: 33g | Fiber: 3g | Protein: 1g | Sodium: 0mg | Vitamin A: 2% DV | Vitamin C: 25% DV

12. Berry Kombucha Drink

Preparation Time: 5 Minutes | Serves: 2

Ingredients:

- 1 cup frozen mixed berries
- ½ cup Bill's Strawberry Kefir

- 1 cup Cranberry Ginger Kombucha (e.g., GT's Enlightened Organic Raw Cosmic Cranberry)

Directions:

1. Blend frozen berries and kefir until smooth, adding water if needed.
2. Mix with kombucha, pour into glasses, and enjoy immediately or chill for later.

Nutrition Highlights: Calories: 100 | Fat: 1g | Carbs: 20g | Fiber: 2g | Protein: 3g | Vitamin C: 40%

13. Blackberry Green Tea & Lemonade

Preparation Time: 5 Minutes | Serves: 2

Ingredients:

- 1 cup Water Kefir
- ½ cup chilled brewed green tea
- 3 tablespoons fresh lemon juice
- 2 teaspoons granulated sugar
- ½ cup fresh blackberries
- 8-10 ice cubes
- 2 fresh lemon slices for garnish

Directions:

1. Combine kefir, green tea, lemon juice, and sugar.
2. Divide blackberries and ice between glasses, pour mixture over, and garnish with lemon.

Nutrition Highlights: Calories: 60 | Carbs: 16g | Fiber: 3g | Protein: 1g | Vitamin C: 40%

14. Creamy Blueberry Pomegranate Smoothie

Preparation Time: 5 Minutes | Serves: 1

Ingredients:

- ½ cup fresh blueberries
- ½ cup 100% blueberry pomegranate juice
- 4 ice cubes
- ½ cup Apple Ginger Kefir

Directions:

1. Blend blueberries, pomegranate juice, and ice until smooth.
2. Mix with kefir in a glass, stir, and serve chilled.

Nutrition Highlights: Calories: 190 | Fat: 1.5g | Carbs: 43g | Fiber: 3g | Protein: 4g | Vitamin C: 20%

15. Mocha Kefir Delight

Preparation Time: 5 Minutes | Serves: 2

Ingredients:

- ¾ cup chilled brewed coffee
- ½ cup plain kefir
- 1 tablespoon agave nectar
- 1 tablespoon homemade dark chocolate sauce
- 1½ teaspoons unsweetened cocoa powder
- 1 teaspoon vanilla extract

Directions:

1. Blend all ingredients until smooth and frothy.
2. Pour into glasses and enjoy a chocolaty energy boost.

Nutrition Highlights: Calories: 110 | Fat: 2g | Carbs: 21g | Fiber: 2g | Protein: 4g | Calcium: 8%

16. Ginger Freeze

Preparation Time: 2 Minutes | Serves: 1

Ingredients:

- 8 ounces of club soda
- 4-6 Ginger Beer ice cubes

Directions:

1. Mix club soda with Ginger Beer ice cubes in a glass and serve for an instant refresh.

Nutrition Highlights: Calories: 50 | Carbs: 12g

17. Pineapple Chia Kefir Colada

Preparation Time: 5 Minutes | Serves: 2

Ingredients:

- 1 cup fresh pineapple cubes
- ½ cup light coconut milk
- ½ cup plain kefir
- 2 teaspoons chia seeds

Directions:

1. Blend all ingredients until smooth.

2. Divide into glasses and serve as a tropical energizer.

Nutrition Highlights: Calories: 255 | Fat: 8g | Carbs: 44g | Fiber: 6g | Protein: 5g | Vitamin C: 120%

18.   Miso Sunrise

Preparation Time: 5 Minutes | Serves: 2

Ingredients:

- 2-3 chopped kale leaves
- 1 chopped carrot or ¼ cup 100% carrot juice
- 2 cups cold water
- 2 teaspoons organic mellow white miso
- 2 teaspoons minced fresh ginger
- 1 teaspoon tamari
- ¼ teaspoon garlic powder

Directions:

1. Blend all ingredients until smooth.
2. Serve immediately or chill to refresh later, enjoying a savory twist on your morning.

Nutrition Highlights: Calories: 50 | Carbs: 10g | Fiber: 2g | Protein: 3g | Vitamin A: 220% | Vitamin C: 70%

19.   Lemon Freeze

Preparation Time: 5 Minutes | Serves: 2

Ingredients:

- 1 cup Probiotic Lemonade
- 20 ice cubes (about 2 cups)
- 2 lemon slices for garnish

Directions:

1. Blend lemonade and ice until smooth.
2. Garnish with lemon slices, serve chilled, and rejuvenate your day.

Nutrition Highlights: Calories: 50 | Carbs: 15g | Fiber: 2g | Vitamin C: 40%

20.   Creamy Iced Chai

Preparation Time: 2 Minutes | Serves: 1

Ingredients:

- ½ cup chai tea concentrate
- ½ cup plain kefir
- 3-4 ice cubes

Directions:

1. Whisk chai concentrate and kefir, add ice, stir, and enjoy a flavorful energy boost.

Nutrition Highlights: Calories: 150 | Fat: 1g | Carbs: 28g | Protein: 6g | Calcium: 15%

21.   Double Cherry Kombucha

Preparation Time: 5 Minutes | Serves: 1

Ingredients:

- 1 cup frozen dark sweet cherries
- ½ cup tart cherry juice
- ½ cup Original Kombucha
- 1 teaspoon agave nectar (optional)

Directions:

1. Blend cherries and juice until smooth.

2. Stir into kombucha, adjust sweetness with agave if needed, and savor the cherry delight.

Nutrition Highlights: Calories: 180 | Carbs: 42g | Fiber: 3g | Protein: 2g | Vitamin C: 15%

22. Chocolate Espresso Bean Kefir

Preparation Time: 5 Minutes | Serves: 2

Ingredients:

- ½ cup chilled brewed coffee
- ½ cup plain kefir
- ½ cup light almond milk
- 1½ tablespoons homemade dark chocolate sauce
- 9 chocolate-covered espresso beans or 1 shot of espresso
- 5-6 ice cubes

Directions:

1. Blend all ingredients until frothy.

2. Enjoy a creamy, caffeinated treat perfect for any coffee lover.

Nutrition Highlights: Calories: 90 | Fat: 3.5g | Carbs: 13g | Protein: 4g | Calcium: 20%

23. Hemp Shake

Preparation Time: 5 Minutes | Serves: 2

Ingredients:

- ¾ cup plain cultured almond milk yogurt or 1 banana
- ½ cup light almond milk
- 1 tablespoon hemp powder
- 4-5 ice cubes
- 2 teaspoons honey (optional)

Directions:

1. Combine all ingredients, and blend until smooth.

2. Divide into glasses, offering a nutrient-packed start to the day.

Nutrition Highlights: Calories: 150 | Fat: 2.5g | Carbs: 31g | Fiber: 4g | Protein: 3g | Magnesium: 13%

24. Probiotic Lemonade

Preparation Time: 5 Minutes | Serves: 4

Ingredients:

- 1 quart Water Kefir
- ¼ cup fresh lemon juice
- 1 sliced and seeded lemon

Directions:

1. Mix kefir, lemon juice, and lemon slices.

2. Serve over ice or chilled, refreshing with every sip.

Nutrition Highlights: Calories: 50 | Carbs: 15g | Fiber: 2g | Vitamin C: 40%

25. Mocha Shake

Preparation Time: 5 Minutes | Serves: 1

Ingredients:

- ½ cup vanilla nonfat frozen yogurt (live cultures)
- ½ cup chilled brewed coffee
- 1½ teaspoons unsweetened cocoa powder

Directions:

1. Blend all ingredients until smooth.

2. Serve as a delightful alternative to your regular coffee routine.

Nutrition Highlights: Calories: 110 | Carbs: 21g | Protein: 5g | Calcium: 15%

26. Apple Ginger Kefir Bliss

Preparation Time: 5 Minutes | Total Time: 5 Minutes | Serves: 2

Ingredients*:*

- 1 Honeycrisp apple, quartered and cored
- ½ cup Traditional Plain Kefir or plain kefir
- ½ cup Homemade Almond Milk or light almond milk
- 1 teaspoon fresh ginger, finely chopped
- 1½ teaspoons organic coconut palm sugar
- 4 to 5 ice cubes

Directions:

1. In a high-speed blender, combine the apple, kefir, almond milk, and ginger until smooth.

2. Add the coconut palm sugar and ice cubes, blending until you achieve a frothy texture.

3. Pour into two glasses and enjoy immediately or refrigerate for up to 3-4 days.

Nutrition per serving*:* 140 Calories | Fat 2g | Saturated Fat 1g | Sodium 140mg | Carbs 26g | Fiber 3g | Sugars 23g | Protein 6g

27. Spiced Apple Kombucha Delight

Preparation Time: 10 Minutes | Total Time: 40 Minutes | Serves: 2

Ingredients:

- 1 apple, cored and sliced
- 1 cup GT's Enlightened Organic Raw Original Kombucha or similar
- ¼ cup Oregon Chai Tea Concentrate or 1 teaspoon chai tea spice
- 6 ice cubes

Directions:

1. Place apple slices and kombucha in two glasses, allowing them to infuse for 20-30 minutes.

2. Remove apple slices, then stir in the chai tea concentrate or spice.

3. Add ice cubes and serve immediately or refrigerate for up to 3-4 days.

Nutrition per serving*:* 80 Calories | Fat 0g | Sodium 20mg | Carbs 20g | Fiber 1g | Sugars 13g | Protein 0g

28. Tart Cherry Kefir Antioxidant

Preparation Time: 5 Minutes | Total Time: 5 Minutes | Serves: 2

Ingredients:

- 1 cup frozen dark cherries
- ½ cup plain kefir or Traditional Plain Kefir
- ½ cup 100% tart cherry juice
- 4 to 5 ice cubes

Directions:

1. Blend all ingredients until smooth and icy.
2. Serve in two glasses or keep chilled for 3-4 days.

Nutrition per serving: 110 Calories | Fat 0.5g | Sodium 40mg | Carbs 22g | Fiber 2g | Sugars 18g | Protein 4g

29. Chocolate Cherry Smoothie for the Soul

Preparation Time: 5 Minutes | Total Time: 5 Minutes | Serves: 2

Ingredients:

- 3 ounces silken tofu (about ⅓ block)
- ¼ cup nonfat plain Greek yogurt
- 1 tablespoon unsweetened cocoa powder
- 1 banana
- ½ cup tart cherry juice

Directions:

1. Combine tofu, yogurt, and cocoa in a blender until smooth.
2. Add banana and cherry juice, blending again to perfection.
3. Pour into two glasses and savor or refrigerate to enjoy later.

Nutrition per serving: 130 Calories | Fat 1.5g | Sodium 25mg | Carbs 25g | Fiber 2g | Sugars 15g | Protein 6g

30. Cinnamon Swirl Raisin Delight

Preparation Time: 5 Minutes | Total Time: 5 Minutes | Serves: 2

Ingredients:

- 1 cup low-fat or nonfat plain yogurt or ½ cup low-fat or nonfat milk
- ½ cup raisins
- ½ cup chilled, cooked brown rice
- 1 teaspoon ground cinnamon
- 4 to 5 ice cubes

Directions:

1. Blend yogurt (or milk), raisins, brown rice, and cinnamon until smooth.
2. Add ice cubes and blend again until silky.
3. Enjoy immediately in two glasses or chill for later delight.

Nutrition per serving: 160 Calories | Fat 1.5g | Sodium 90mg | Carbs 26g | Fiber 2g | Sugars 11g | Protein 11g

31. Banana Papaya Smoothie

Preparation Time: 5 Minutes | Total Time: 5 Minutes | Serves: 2

Ingredients:

- 1 banana
- 1 cup cubed papaya
- ½ cup Water Kefir
- 4 to 5 ice cubes

Directions:

1. Combine banana, papaya, water kefir, and ice in a blender until creamy.

2. Serve this tropical concoction in two glasses or keep it cool for an anytime treat.

Nutrition per serving: 100 Calories | Fat 0g | Sodium 5mg | Carbs 24g | Fiber 3g | Sugars 15g | Protein 1g

32. Cranberry Ginger Kombucha Fusion

Preparation Time: 5 Minutes | Total Time: 5 Minutes | Serves: 1

Ingredients:

- ½ cup GT's Enlightened Organic Raw Original Kombucha or similar
- ½ cup frozen whole cranberries
- 1 teaspoon chopped fresh ginger

Directions:

1. Blend kombucha, cranberries, and ginger until smooth, adding water if needed.

2. Enjoy this refreshing blend immediately or store it chilled for a burst of energy.

Nutrition per serving: 60 Calories | Fat 0g | Sodium 5mg | Carbs 15g | Fiber 4g | Sugars 5g | Protein 0g

33. Creamy Blackberry Probiotic Smoothie

Preparation Time: 5 Minutes | Total Time: 5 Minutes | Serves: 1

Ingredients:

- 1 cup fresh blackberries
- ½ cup low-fat buttermilk
- 1 teaspoon honey

Directions:

1. Combine blackberries, buttermilk, and honey in a blender until smooth.

2. Savor the natural goodness immediately or keep it in the fridge for a later health boost.

Nutrition per serving: 130 Calories | Fat 2g | Sodium 130mg | Carbs 25g | Fiber 8g | Sugars 19g | Protein 6g

34. Go Bananas Potassium Rich Smoothie

Preparation Time: 5 Minutes | Total Time: 5 Minutes | Serves: 2

Ingredients:

- 2 frozen bananas
- 1 cup low-fat or nonfat milk
- ½ cup Walnut Honey Kefir

Directions:

1. Puree bananas, milk, and kefir until you achieve a creamy, dreamy consistency.

2. Divide this potassium-packed treat between two glasses or store it for a nutritious snack.

Nutrition per serving: 160 Calories | Fat 3.5g | Sodium 120mg | Carbs 31g | Fiber 4g | Sugars 24g | Protein 17g

35. Honey Almond Antioxidant Shake

Preparation Time: 5 Minutes | Total Time: 5 Minutes | Serves: 2

Ingredients:

- 1 cup low-fat or nonfat plain yogurt or ¼ cup light almond milk
- 2 tablespoons almond cream
- 1 to 2 tablespoons dark honey
- 8 ice cubes

Directions:

1. Blend yogurt (or almond milk), almond cream, and honey until frothy.

2. Pour into glasses for a sweet, antioxidant-rich indulgence, or refrigerate to enjoy anytime.

Nutrition per serving: 130 Calories | Fat 4g | Sodium 100mg | Carbs 19g | Sugars 18g | Protein 6g

36. Acai Melon Refresher

Preparation Time: 5 Minutes | Total Time: 5 Minutes | Serves: 2

Ingredients:

- 2 cups fresh watermelon, cubed
- ½ cup acai berry juice (e.g., R.W. Knudsen Family Organic)
- ½ cup low-fat or nonfat plain yogurt or Homemade Yogurt
- 4 to 5 ice cubes

Directions:

1. Blend watermelon, acai berry juice, and yogurt until perfectly smooth.

2. Add ice cubes and blend again for a chilled, refreshing shake.

3. Serve immediately in two glasses or refrigerate for a quick, energizing drink later.

Nutrition per serving: 100 Calories | Fat 0g | Sodium 30mg | Carbs 20g | Fiber <1g | Sugars 17g | Protein 7g

37. Papaya Kefir Sunrise

Preparation Time: 5 Minutes | Total Time: 5 Minutes | Serves: 1

Ingredients:

- 1 cup fresh papaya, cubed
- ¾ cup Pineapple Chia Colada Kefir or Lifeway Coconut-Chia Kefir
- 4 to 5 ice cubes

Directions:

1. Combine papaya and kefir in a blender, and blend until smooth.
2. Add ice and blend until you reach a frosty consistency.
3. Pour into a glass and enjoy this sunny, nutritious delight, or store it for up to 3-4 days.

Nutrition per serving: 150 Calories | Fat 4.5g | Sodium 35mg | Carbs 25g | Fiber 5g | Sugars 17g | Protein 4g

38. Pom-Pineapple Kombucha Fizz

Preparation Time: 5 Minutes | Total Time: 5 Minutes | Serves: 2

Ingredients:

- 1 cup frozen pineapple
- ½ cup 100% pomegranate juice (e.g., POM Wonderful)
- ½ cup Original Kombucha or GT's Enlightened Organic Raw Original Kombucha
- 1 teaspoon agave nectar (optional)

Directions:

1. Blend pineapple and pomegranate juice until smooth, adding water if needed.
2. Mix in kombucha and agave nectar for a hint of sweetness if desired.
3. Serve this fizzy, fruity concoction in two glasses, or keep chilled for a refreshing boost anytime.

Nutrition per serving: 90 Calories | Fat 0g | Sodium 5mg | Carbs 22g | Fiber 1g | Sugars 17g | Protein 0g

39. Pumpkin Spice Kefir Smoothie

Preparation Time: 5 Minutes | Total Time: 5 Minutes | Serves: 2

Ingredients:

- 1 cup Vanilla Bean Smoothie
- ½ cup canned pumpkin puree
- ½ cup cashew cream
- 1 tablespoon pure maple syrup
- ¼ teaspoon ground cinnamon
- 4 to 5 ice cubes

Directions:

1. Blend vanilla smoothie, pumpkin puree, cashew cream, maple syrup, and cinnamon until smooth.
2. Add ice to achieve a creamy texture, akin to pumpkin pie in a glass.

3. Enjoy this autumn-inspired treat in two glasses or refrigerate it to savor the flavors later.

Nutrition per serving: 210 Calories | Fat 9g | Sodium 45mg | Carbs 25g | Fiber 3g | Sugars 16g | Protein 10g

40. Purple Power Antioxidant Shake

Preparation Time: 5 Minutes | Total Time: 5 Minutes | Serves: 2

Ingredients:

- 1 cup frozen sweet dark cherries
- ½ cup Traditional Plain Kefir or plain filmjölk
- ½ cup 100% grape juice
- 1 tablespoon acai powder

Directions:

1. Combine cherries, kefir, grape juice, and acai powder in a blender for a nutrient-packed blend.

2. Serve this deeply colored, antioxidant-rich shake in two glasses, or keep chilled for a healthful pick-me-up.

Nutrition per serving: 120 Calories | Fat 1g | Sodium 35mg | Carbs 25g | Fiber 2g | Sugars 22g | Protein 3g

41. Roasted Apple Smoothie

Preparation Time: 25 Minutes | Total Time: 30 Minutes | Serves: 2

Ingredients:

- 1 cup Vanilla Bean Smoothie

- ½ cup low-fat or nonfat milk
- ½ cup roasted cinnamon apples
- 1 apple, with peel, cored and sliced
- 4 to 5 ice cubes

Directions:

1. Roast sliced apples with cinnamon until tender, let cool.

2. Blend vanilla smoothie, milk, and cooled roasted apples until creamy.

3. Add fresh apple slices and ice, blending until smooth.

4. Divide this orchard-inspired smoothie between two glasses or refrigerate for a cozy treat later.

Nutrition per serving: 140 Calories | Fat 1.5g | Sodium 85mg | Carbs 28g | Fiber 4g | Sugars 22g | Protein 6g

42. Vanilla Bean Dream Smoothie

Preparation Time: 10 Minutes | Total Time: 10 Minutes | Serves: 3

Ingredients:

- 1½ vanilla bean pods
- 1 cup Traditional Plain Kefir or filmjölk
- 1 cup low-fat or nonfat plain Greek yogurt
- 2 tablespoons agave nectar
- 8 ice cubes

Directions:

1. Scrape seeds from vanilla pods and blend with kefir, yogurt, and agave nectar.

2. Add ice, blending until smooth and dreamy.

3. Serve this vanilla bean-speckled delight in three glasses or keep chilled for a luxurious treat.

Nutrition per serving: 110 Calories | Fat 0.5g | Sodium 75mg | Carbs 14g | Sugars 14g | Protein 12g

43. Walnut Honey Kefir Smoothie

Preparation Time: 5 Minutes | Total Time: 5 Minutes | Serves: 2

Ingredients:

- 1 cup Traditional Plain Kefir
- ½ cup walnuts
- ½ cup low-fat or nonfat milk
- 2 teaspoons honey
- 4 to 5 ice cubes

Directions:

1. Blend kefir, walnuts, milk, and honey until perfectly combined.

2. Add ice and blend into a smooth, nutty concoction.

3. Pour this omega-3-rich smoothie into two glasses or store it for a nourishing snack anytime.

Nutrition per serving: 320 Calories | Fat 18g | Sodium 90mg | Carbs 29g | Fiber 2g | Sugars 27g | Protein 14g

44. Raspberry-Ginger Slush

Preparation Time: 5 Minutes | Total Time: 5 Minutes | Serves: 2

Ingredients:

- 1 cup frozen raspberries
- 1 cup Ginger Beer (homemade or store-bought)
- ½ cup water

Directions:

1. Blend raspberries, ginger beer, and water until you achieve an icy, smooth consistency.

2. Pour into two glasses for a refreshing detox boost.

Nutrition per serving: 90 Calories | Fat 0g | Sodium 0mg | Carbs 23g | Fiber 2g | Sugars 20g | Protein <1g

45. Cantaloupe Lassi Miracle

Preparation Time: 5 Minutes | Total Time: 5 Minutes | Serves: 1

Ingredients:

- 1 cup Vanilla Lassi or Vanilla Bean Smoothie
- 1 cup cubed cantaloupe
- 4 to 5 ice cubes

Directions:

1. Combine lassi, cantaloupe, and ice in a blender until frothy and smooth.

2. Serve this vitamin A-rich drink for a nutritious start or end to your day.

Nutrition per serving: 190 Calories | Fat 3.5g | Sodium 160mg | Carbs 33g | Fiber 3g | Sugars 31g | Protein 9g

46. Cherry Lime Fizz Refresher

Preparation Time: 5 Minutes | Total Time: 5 Minutes | Serves: 1

Ingredients:

- 1 cup frozen dark sweet cherries
- 2 tablespoons fresh lime juice
- 1 teaspoon agave nectar (optional)
- ¼ cup Ginger Kombucha or similar

Directions:

1. Puree cherries and lime juice, adding water as needed. Sweeten with agave if desired.
2. Stir in kombucha for a fizzy, detoxifying treat.

Nutrition per serving: 110 Calories | Fat 0g | Sodium 0mg | Carbs 26g | Fiber 3g | Sugars 19g | Protein 1g

47. Cran-Lemon Basil Smoothie

Preparation Time: 5 Minutes | Total Time: 5 Minutes | Serves: 2

Ingredients:

- 1 cup frozen whole cranberries
- 1 cup Probiotic Lemonade

- ¼ cup 100% orange juice
- 4 fresh basil leaves
- 1 teaspoon honey (optional)
- 1 lemon slice, halved for garnish

Directions:

1. Blend cranberries, lemonade, orange juice, and basil until smooth. Sweeten with honey if needed.
2. Garnish with a lemon slice for a detox delight.

Nutrition per serving: 60 Calories | Fat 0g | Sodium 5mg | Carbs 16g | Fiber 3g | Sugars 9g | Protein <1g

48. Cucumber Mint Freshness

Preparation Time: 5 Minutes | Total Time: 5 Minutes | Serves: 2

Ingredients:

- 1 cup plain low-fat or nonfat yogurt (or Homemade Yogurt)
- 1 cup cubed cucumber
- 2 tablespoons fresh mint
- 1 tablespoon fresh lemon juice
- 1 teaspoon garlic powder

Directions:

1. Blend yogurt, cucumber, mint, lemon juice, and garlic powder until smooth for a tzatziki-inspired smoothie.
2. Enjoy this refreshing, protein-boosted beverage.

Nutrition per serving: 80 Calories | Fat 1.5g | Sodium 80mg | Carbs 12g | Sugars 9g | Protein 6g

49. Creamy Tomato Smoothie

Preparation Time: 5 Minutes | Total Time: 5 Minutes | Serves: 1

Ingredients:

- ½ cup tomato juice (choose low-sodium for a healthier option)
- ½ cup chopped seeded unpeeled cucumber
- ¼ cup plain kefir or Traditional Plain Kefir

Directions:

1. Blend tomato juice, cucumber, and kefir until you have a smooth, creamy concoction.
2. Enjoy this veggie-packed smoothie, a perfect kickstart for your morning detox.

Nutrition per serving: 90 Calories | Fat 1g | Sodium 400mg | Carbs 13g | Fiber 1g | Sugars 10g | Protein 7g

50. Green Goodness Smoothie

Preparation Time: 5 Minutes | Total Time: 5 Minutes | Serves: 1

Ingredients:

- ½ cup stemmed kale
- ½ cup apple cider
- ½ apple, cored
- 2 strawberries, hulled
- ½ cup vanilla bean Greek yogurt

Directions:

1. Combine kale, cider, apple, and strawberries in a blender until smooth.
2. Mix with vanilla yogurt for a sweet, nutrient-rich green drink.

Nutrition per serving: 250 Calories | Fat 2.5g | Sodium 75mg | Carbs 48g | Fiber 3g | Sugars 37g | Protein 10g

51. Grapefruit Ginger Fizz

Preparation Time: 5 Minutes | Total Time: 5 Minutes | Serves: 1

Ingredients:

- ½ medium grapefruit peeled and roughly chopped
- 1 cup Ginger Beer (homemade or store-bought)
- 2 or 3 ice cubes

Directions:

1. Crush grapefruit with ginger beer until smooth. Serve over ice for a tangy, revitalizing drink.
2. This beverage is a vitamin C powerhouse, perfect for immune support and detox.

Nutrition per serving: 140 Calories | Fat 0g | Sodium 0mg | Carbs 35g | Fiber 1g | Sugars 34g | Protein <1g

52. Cran-Apple Ginger Freeze

Preparation Time: 5 Minutes | Total Time: 5 Minutes | Serves: 2

Ingredients:

- 1 apple, cored
- 1 cup Ginger Beer (homemade or store-bought)
- ½ cup frozen whole cranberries

Directions*:*

1. Blend apple, ginger beer, and cranberries until icy and smooth.
2. Share this fiber-rich, refreshing freeze with a friend, or enjoy it all by yourself.

Nutrition per serving*:* 100 Calories | Fat 0g | Sodium 0mg | Carbs 26g | Fiber 3g | Sugars 21g | Protein 0g

53. Lemon-Lime Kefir Water

Preparation Time: 5 Minutes | Total Time: 5 Minutes | Serves: 1

Ingredients:

- 3 fresh lime slices
- 2 fresh lemon slices
- ½ cup Water Kefir
- 4 or 5 ice cubes

Directions:

1. Muddle lime and lemon slices in a glass, then add kefir and ice for a citrus-infused probiotic drink.

2. A perfect hydrating beverage to help with detox and digestion.

Nutrition per serving: 45 Calories | Fat 0g | Sodium 10mg | Carbs 12g | Fiber 2g | Sugars 9g | Protein <1g

54. Miso Tomato Smoothie

Preparation Time: 5 Minutes | Total Time: 5 Minutes | Serves: 1

Ingredients:

- 1 cup cherry tomatoes
- ½ cup vegetable broth (opt for low-sodium)
- ½ cup 100% carrot juice
- 1 teaspoon organic mellow white miso

Directions*:*

1. Blend tomatoes, broth, carrot juice, and miso until smooth for a zesty, savory treat.
2. This smoothie is a vitamin A goldmine, offering a daily boost in a single serving.

Nutrition per serving*:* 80 Calories | Fat 0.5g | Sodium 500mg | Carbs 16g | Fiber 3g | Sugars 11g | Protein 2g

55. Pear Raspberry Smoothie

Preparation Time: 5 Minutes | Total Time: 5 Minutes | Serves: 3

Ingredients:

- 1 container (5.3 ounces) low-fat or nonfat pear Greek yogurt (or substitute with vanilla Greek yogurt)

- 1 cup frozen raspberries

- 1 cup low-fat or nonfat milk

- 1 pear, quartered and cored

Directions:

1. Blend yogurt, raspberries, milk, and pear until silky smooth.

2. This high-fiber smoothie is ideal for a filling breakfast or a satisfying snack.

Nutrition per serving: 130 Calories | Fat 1.5g | Sodium 55mg | Carbs 25g | Fiber 6g | Sugars 18g | Protein 8g

56. Peach Ginger Kombucha Splash

Preparation Time: 5 Minutes | Total Time: 5 Minutes | Serves: 1

Ingredients:

- 1 cup frozen peach slices (or fresh peaches if available)

- ¼ cup water

- 1 teaspoon honey

- ½ cup Ginger Kombucha or similar

Directions:

1. Puree peaches, water, and honey until smooth.

2. Stir into kombucha for a sweet, tangy refreshment with a ginger twist.

Nutrition per serving: 100 Calories | Fat 0g | Sodium 5mg | Carbs 25g | Fiber 3g | Sugars 21g | Protein 2g

57. Pineapple Cucumber Cool Down

Preparation Time: 5 Minutes | Total Time: 5 Minutes | Serves: 2

Ingredients:

- 1 cup low-fat or nonfat vanilla yogurt

- 1 cup sliced cucumber

- ½ cup cubed fresh pineapple

Directions:

1. Blend yogurt, cucumber, and pineapple until you achieve a creamy, smooth texture.

2. Dive into this hydrating, digestive-friendly smoothie for a mid-day refresh.

Nutrition per serving: 150 Calories | Fat 2g | Sodium 60mg | Carbs 24g | Fiber <1g | Sugars 18g | Protein 9g

58. Purple Kombucha Power

Preparation Time: 5 Minutes | Total Time: 5 Minutes | Serves: 1

Ingredients:

- ½ cup blueberries

- ½ cup 100% pomegranate juice

- 4 ice cubes

- ½ cup Ginger Kombucha or similar

Directions:

1. Blend blueberries, pomegranate juice, and ice until icy and smooth.

2. Stir in kombucha for an antioxidant-rich, vibrant drink.

Nutrition per serving: 120 Calories | Fat 0g | Sodium 10mg | Carbs 31g | Fiber 62g | Sugars 22g | Protein <1g

59. Red Dragon Beet Smoothie

Preparation Time: 5 Minutes | Total Time: 5 Minutes | Serves: 1

Ingredients:

- ½ cup chilled roasted chopped beets

- ½ cup low-fat or nonfat plain Greek yogurt

- ½ cup pomegranate juice

- 1 teaspoon fresh chopped ginger

Directions:

1. Combine roasted beets, yogurt, pomegranate juice, and ginger until smooth.

2. Revel in the earthy flavors and health benefits of this deep red tonic.

Nutrition per serving: 170 Calories | Fat 0g | Sodium 125mg | Carbs 30g | Fiber 2g | Sugars 25g | Protein 13g

60. Half And Half Tea Refresh

Preparation Time: 5 Minutes | Total Time: 5 Minutes | Serves: 2

Ingredients:

- 1 cup water

- 1 tablespoon fresh lemon juice

- 1 teaspoon sugar

- ½ cup Original Kombucha or similar

- 4 or 5 ice cubes

Directions:

1. Stir water, lemon juice, and sugar until sugar dissolves. Mix in kombucha and ice.

2. Enjoy this probiotic-rich, lightly sweetened twist on a classic half-and-half tea.

Nutrition per serving: 15 Calories | Fat 0g | Sodium 0mg | Carbs 4g | Fiber 0g | Sugars 3g | Protein 0g

61. Ginger Kombucha Zest

Preparation Time: 1-2 Hours (for steeping) | Total Time: 2 Hours | Serves: 2

Ingredients:

- 1 cup Original Kombucha or similar

- 2 teaspoons minced fresh ginger

- 6 ice cubes

Directions:

1. Steep kombucha with minced ginger for 1-2 hours (or overnight in the fridge for stronger flavor).

2. Strain, then serve over ice for a spicy, digestive-aiding beverage.

Nutrition per serving: 35 Calories | Fat 0g | Sodium 10mg | Carbs 8g | Fiber 0g | Sugars 2g | Protein 0g

62.   Berry Beet Vitamin C Boost

Prep Time: 5 Minutes | Total Time: 5 Minutes | Serves: 1

Ingredients:

- 1 cup Traditional Plain Kefir or plain kefir
- 1 cup strawberries, sliced
- 1 small beet (~1½ inches diameter), peeled
- 1-2 tsp agave nectar (optional)

Directions:

1. Blend kefir, strawberries, and beet until silky smooth in a high-speed blender. For sweetness, add agave to taste.

2. Enjoy fresh or refrigerate for a vitamin-packed treat for up to 3-4 days.

Nutrition per serving: Calories 190 | Fat 2.5g | Sodium 190mg | Carbs 31g | Fiber 5g | Sugars 24g | Protein 13g

63.   Banana Berry B Vitamin Fusion

Prep Time: 5 Minutes | Total Time: 5 Minutes | Serves: 1

Ingredients:

- 2 oz tempeh
- ½ banana
- 4-5 strawberries, hulled
- ½ cup Homemade Almond Milk or light almond milk
- ¼ cup 100% orange juice
- 1 tsp agave nectar
- 4-5 ice cubes

Directions:

1. Combine all ingredients in a blender until perfectly blended.

2. Serve immediately for a B-vitamin boost, or keep chilled for up to 3-4 days.

Nutrition per serving: Calories 260 | Fat 3.5g | Sodium 75mg | Carbs 47g | Fiber 4g | Sugars 28g | Protein 13g

64.   Berry Green Probiotic Twist

Prep Time: 5 Minutes | Total Time: 5 Minutes | Serves: 1

Ingredients:

- 1 cup baby spinach, stemmed
- 4 large strawberries, fresh and hulled
- ½ cup Probiotic Lemonade
- 1 cup strawberries, frozen

Directions:

1. Smooth blend of spinach, fresh strawberries, and lemonade. Add

frozen strawberries for a frosty finish.

2. Sip fresh or store in the fridge, indulging in probiotics and vitamins for days.

Nutrition per serving: Calories 140 | Fat 1g | Sodium 15mg | Carbs 36g | Fiber 8g | Sugars 22g | Protein 3g

65. Butternut Squash Vitamin A Gold

Prep Time: 7 Minutes | Total Time: 32 Minutes | Serves: 1

Ingredients:

- ½ cup sliced leeks
- 1 cup roasted butternut squash, chilled
- 1 cup vegetable broth
- 1 tsp organic mellow white miso
- ¼ tsp garlic powder
- ⅛ tsp sea salt

Directions:

1. Sauté leeks in a dry pan until tender. Blend with squash, broth, miso, and spices until creamy.

2. Enjoy a burst of vitamin A fresh or keep it cool for later.

Nutrition per serving: Calories 120 | Fat 0.5g | Sodium 620mg | Carbs 29g | Fiber 4g | Sugars 6g | Protein 3g

66. Silky Coco-Cado Antioxidant Dream

Prep Time: 5 Minutes | Total Time: 5 Minutes | Serves: 2

Ingredients:

- 1½ cups unsweetened coconut milk beverage
- 1 avocado, pitted and peeled
- 1 tbsp unsweetened cocoa powder
- 1 tbsp agave nectar

Directions:

1. Smoothly blend coconut milk and avocado. Mix in cocoa and agave for a silky sip.

2. Divide and delight in or chill for a taste of antioxidants at any time.

Nutrition per serving: Calories 200 | Fat 17g | Sodium 20mg | Carbs 16g | Fiber 8g | Sugars 6g | Protein 2g

67. Veggie Patch Creamy Delight

Prep Time: 5 Minutes | Total Time: 5 Minutes | Serves: 2

Ingredients:

- 1 cup Homemade Almond Milk or light almond milk
- ½ cup sweet potato puree
- ½ cup frozen vanilla yogurt
- ½ cup each of frozen peaches, mango, and butternut squash

- 1 tbsp agave nectar

Directions:

1. Blend all for a thick, creamy treat. Thin as desired with water or milk.

2. Enjoy a creamy dose of beta-carotene now or keep chilled for later.

Nutrition per serving: Calories 230 | Fat 3g | Sodium 135mg | Carbs 49g | Fiber 3g | Sugars 31g | Protein 5g

68. Sweet Potato Protein Pack

Prep Time: 5 Minutes | Total Time: 5 Minutes | Serves: 2

Ingredients:

- 1 cup sweet potato puree
- ½ cup Homemade Yogurt or low-fat yogurt
- ¼ cup apple cider
- 1 scoop vanilla protein powder
- 4-5 ice cubes

Directions:

1. Combine sweet potato, yogurt, cider, and protein powder in a blender until smooth.

2. Enjoy a protein and vitamin A-rich smoothie immediately or store it for a nutritious snack.

Nutrition per serving: Calories 200 | Fat 1.5g | Sodium 170mg | Carbs 37g | Fiber 3g | Sugars 14g | Protein 10g

69. Coconut Strawberry Whip

Prep Time: 5 Minutes | Total Time: 5 Minutes | Serves: 1

Ingredients:

- ¾ cup cultured coconut milk, strawberry-flavored
- ½ cup light coconut milk
- ½ cup fresh raspberries

Directions:

1. Blend cultured coconut milk, light coconut milk, and raspberries until smooth and creamy.

2. Savor the silky texture and vibrant flavors immediately or refrigerate to indulge later.

Nutrition per serving: Calories 240 | Fat 15g | Saturated Fat 12g | Sodium 30mg | Carbs 27g | Fiber 8g | Sugars 17g | Protein <1g

70. Very Veggie Kefir Revitalizer

Prep Time: 5 Minutes | Total Time: 5 Minutes | Serves: 3

Ingredients:

- 1 stalk rainbow chard, chopped (about 1½ cups)
- 1 medium stalk celery, chopped
- ½ cup cucumber, chopped

- ½ cup plain kefir or Traditional Plain Kefir
- ½ cup Homemade Almond Milk or light almond milk
- 1 avocado, pitted and peeled
- ½ cup 100% white grape juice
- ½ cup water
- ⅛ tsp sea salt

Directions:

1. Combine chard, celery, cucumber, kefir, and almond milk in a blender until smooth. Blend in avocado, grape juice, water, and salt.

2. Divide among glasses for a vibrant veggie boost or keep refrigerated for up to 3-4 days.

Nutrition per serving: Calories 180 | Fat 10g | Sodium 250mg | Carbs 18g | Fiber 5g | Sugars 13g | Protein 5g

71. Avocado Coconut Freeze

Prep Time: 5 Minutes | Total Time: 5 Minutes | Serves: 2

Ingredients:

- 1 banana, frozen
- 1 avocado, pitted and peeled
- 1 cup plain kefir or Traditional Plain Kefir
- ½ cup light coconut milk
- 1 tsp honey
- 1 oz dark chocolate, shaved

Directions:

1. Blend banana, avocado, kefir, coconut milk, and honey until smooth.

2. Serve in glasses, garnish with shaved dark chocolate, and enjoy a decadent, nutrient-packed treat right away.

Nutrition per serving: Calories 380 | Fat 23g | Saturated Fat 8g | Sodium 80mg | Carbs 39g | Fiber 8g | Sugars 24g | Protein 9g

72. Almond Butter And Jelly Smoothie Revival

Preparation Time: 5 Minutes | Total Time: 5 Minutes | Serves: 1

Ingredients:

- 1 cup frozen mixed berries
- ½ cup Homemade Almond Milk
- ½ cup nonfat plain Greek yogurt
- 2 tablespoons almond butter
- 1 tablespoon agave nectar (optional)

Directions:

1. Blend all ingredients until smooth for a post-workout refreshment.

2. Enjoy immediately or refrigerate to savor after your next workout.

Nutrition per serving: 400 Calories | Fat 19g | Saturated Fat 1.5g | Sodium 135mg | Carbs 45g | Fiber 5g | Sugars 34g | Protein 18g

73. Apple Peanut Butter Smoothie Recharge

Preparation Time: 5 Minutes | Total Time: 5 Minutes | Serves: 3

Ingredients:

- ¾ cup cultured almond milk yogurt
- 1 green apple, quartered and cored
- 1 cup Homemade Almond Milk
- 1 tablespoon agave nectar
- 1 tablespoon creamy natural peanut butter
- 4 to 5 ice cubes

Directions:

1. Combine yogurt, apple, and almond milk in a blender for a smooth base.

2. Add agave nectar and peanut butter, blending to incorporate. Finish with ice for a frosty touch.

3. Distribute among three glasses or keep chilled for a post-exercise treat.

Nutrition per serving: 150 Calories | Fat 4.5g | Sodium 80mg | Carbs 25g | Fiber 4g | Sugars 16g | Protein 2g

74. Apricot Protein Blast

Preparation Time: 5 Minutes | Total Time: 5 Minutes | Serves: 1

Ingredients:

- 2 fresh apricots, pitted
- ½ cup low-fat buttermilk
- 1 scoop vanilla protein powder
- 2 to 3 ice cubes

Directions:

1. Puree apricots, buttermilk, and protein powder until smooth for a tangy, sweet recovery drink.

2. Serve freshly blended to kickstart muscle recovery or keep it in the fridge for later.

Nutrition per serving: 150 Calories | Fat 2.5g | Sodium 260mg | Carbs 19g | Fiber 2g | Sugars 14g | Protein 15g

75. Banana Bread Kefir Nostalgia

Preparation Time: 5 Minutes | Total Time: 5 Minutes | Serves: 1

Ingredients:

- 2 frozen bananas
- ½ cup plain kefir
- ¼ cup Homemade Almond Milk
- ½ teaspoon ground cinnamon

Directions:

1. Blend bananas, kefir, almond milk, and cinnamon until smooth, creating a banana bread-flavored treat.

2. Enjoy the comforting taste post-workout or refrigerate for a quick grab-and-go option.

Nutrition per serving: 290 Calories | Fat 2.5g | Sodium 90mg | Carbs 64g | Fiber 7g | Sugars 38g | Protein 10g

76. Banana Protein Blast Recovery

Preparation Time: 5 Minutes | Total Time: 5 Minutes | Serves: 1

Ingredients:

- 2 ounces tempeh
- 1 cup Homemade Almond Milk
- ½ banana
- 1 tablespoon almond butter
- 1 teaspoon agave nectar

Directions:

1. Combine tempeh, almond milk, banana, and almond butter in a blender for a nutrient-packed mix.

2. Blend until smooth, adding agave nectar for a touch of sweetness.

3. Serve immediately for a potent muscle recovery boost or refrigerate for a post-workout treat.

Nutrition per serving: 210 Calories | Fat 5g | Sodium 200mg | Carbs 32g | Fiber 4g | Sugars 13g | Protein 9g

77. Caramel Banana Smoothie Satisfaction

Preparation Time: 5 Minutes | Total Time: 5 Minutes | Serves: 1

Ingredients:

- 2 frozen bananas
- ½ cup nonfat plain yogurt
- ½ cup cashew cream
- 1 tablespoon caramel sauce

Directions:

1. Puree bananas, yogurt, cashew cream, and caramel until creamy.

2. Enjoy this potassium-rich smoothie right after your workout or save it for a later refreshment.

Nutrition per serving: 210 Calories | Fat 5g | Sodium 200mg | Carbs 32g | Fiber 4g | Sugars 13g | Protein 9g

78. Chocolate Banana Smoothie With A Twist

Preparation Time: 5 Minutes | Total Time: 5 Minutes | Serves: 1

Ingredients:

- 1 banana
- ½ cup Vanilla Lassi (or store-bought)
- ½ cup nonfat milk
- 1 tablespoon unsweetened cocoa powder
- A dash of sea salt (about 1/8 teaspoon)

Directions:

1. Blend banana, vanilla lassi, milk, and cocoa powder until smooth.

2. Add a dash of sea salt to replenish minerals lost during sweating.

3. Serve this salty-sweet recovery drink immediately or store it for a quick post-workout refuel.

Nutrition per serving: 240 Calories | Fat 4g | Sodium 410mg | Carbs 46g | Fiber 6g | Sugars 30g | Protein 10g

79. Creamy Blackberry Ginger Smoothie

Preparation Time: 5 Minutes | Total Time: 5 Minutes | Serves: 1

Ingredients:

- ½ cup nonfat plain Greek yogurt
- ½ cup Original Kombucha with blackberry second ferment
- ½ teaspoon vanilla extract
- 1/8 teaspoon ground ginger

Directions:

1. Stir together yogurt and blackberry kombucha. Add vanilla extract and ginger for enhanced flavor.

2. Mix well and serve as a creamy, probiotic-rich refueling option.

3. Enjoy fresh or keep chilled for a post-exercise boost.

Nutrition per serving: 150 Calories | Fat 0g | Sodium 60mg | Carbs 23g | Fiber 4g | Sugars 16g | Protein 13g

80. Rice Pudding Smoothie Dream

Preparation Time: 5 Minutes | Total Time: 5 Minutes | Serves: 2

Ingredients:

- ½ cup chilled cooked brown rice
- ½ cup nonfat vanilla bean yogurt
- ¼ cup raisins
- ½ apple, cored
- ½ cup Homemade Almond Milk
- ¼ cup light coconut milk
- 1½ teaspoons ground cinnamon

Directions:

1. Start with blending rice, yogurt, and raisins until smooth. Add the apple, almond milk, coconut milk, and cinnamon, and blend again to perfection.

2. Pour the creamy concoction into two glasses, serving a taste of comfort in every sip.

3. This smoothie can be enjoyed immediately or stored in the fridge for a delicious post-workout reward.

Nutrition per serving: 260 Calories | Fat 4g | Saturated Fat 2.5g | Sodium 80mg | Carbs 49g | Fiber 4g | Sugars 31g | Protein 6g

81. Pb Granola Smoothie Energy

Preparation Time: 5 Minutes | Total Time: 5 Minutes | Serves: 2

Ingredients:

- 1 banana
- ½ cup Homemade Almond Milk
- ½ cup nonfat plain Greek yogurt
- ½ cup granola (choose a healthy option like KIND Healthy Grains Oats & Honey Clusters)

- 1 tablespoon natural peanut butter

- 1 tablespoon caramel sauce

Directions:

1. Blend banana, almond milk, yogurt, granola, peanut butter, and caramel sauce until smooth. Expect a slight texture from the granola, adding an interesting twist.

2. Split the blend into two glasses for a nutritious boost, ideal for refueling after workouts.

3. Savor immediately for the best texture or refrigerate for a convenient post-exercise refreshment.

Nutrition per serving: 290 Calories | Fat 9g | Saturated Fat 2g | Sodium 110mg | Carbs 43g | Fiber 5g | Sugars 20g | Protein 11g

82. Ants On A Log Smoothie Innovation

Preparation Time: 5 Minutes | Total Time: 5 Minutes | Serves: 2

Ingredients:

- 1 medium stalk celery, chopped

- ½ cup nonfat plain yogurt

- 1¼ cups nonfat milk

- 2 tablespoons natural peanut butter

- ¼ cup raisins

- 1 teaspoon honey

Directions:

1. Blend celery, yogurt, milk, peanut butter, and half the milk until smooth. Add the remaining milk, raisins, and honey, blending again for a smooth finish.

2. Pour into two glasses, optionally garnishing with extra raisins and celery sticks for a playful touch.

3. Enjoy this novel take on a classic snack immediately, or cool it in the fridge for a refreshing post-workout boost.

Nutrition per serving: 220 Calories | Fat 10g | Saturated Fat 2g | Sodium 120mg | Carbs 28g | Fiber 2g | Sugars 24g | Protein 8g

83. Raspberry Granola Smoothie Boost

Preparation Time: 5 Minutes | Total Time: 5 Minutes | Serves: 2

Ingredients:

- 1 cup frozen raspberries

- 1 cup plain coconut milk beverage

- ½ cup Traditional Plain Kefir

- ½ cup raspberry granola (opt for a healthy option like KIND Healthy Grains Raspberry Clusters with Chia Seeds)

- 1 teaspoon coconut palm sugar

Directions:

1. In a blender, combine raspberries, coconut milk, and kefir until you have a smooth base. Add in the

raspberry granola and coconut palm sugar, blending until fully integrated, yet expect a bit of texture from the granola. 2. Distribute the vibrant mixture into two glasses, each serving as a fiber-rich, probiotic-packed fuel source for muscle recovery.

2. This rejuvenating beverage is perfect for immediate consumption or can be chilled for a refreshing post-workout snack.

Nutrition per serving: 190 Calories | Fat 4.5g | Saturated Fat 2.5g | Sodium 70mg | Carbs 33g | Fiber 6g | Sugars 12g | Protein 5g

84. Oatmeal Cookie Smoothie Bliss

Preparation Time: 5 Minutes | Total Time: 5 Minutes | Serves: 2

Ingredients:

- 1 cup Vanilla Bean Smoothie or store-bought vanilla low-fat yogurt
- ¼ cup old-fashioned oats
- ¼ cup raisins
- ½ cup nonfat milk
- ¼ teaspoon ground cinnamon
- 4 to 5 ice cubes

Directions:

1. Blend the Vanilla Bean Smoothie (or yogurt), oats, and raisins until you achieve a smooth but slightly textured base.

2. Add milk, cinnamon, and ice cubes, blending once more to reach a frosty consistency.

3. Serve the delectable smoothie in two glasses, offering the comforting taste of oatmeal cookies in a nutritious, post-workout drink.

Nutrition per serving: 220 Calories | Fat 2.5g | Saturated Fat 1g | Sodium 70mg | Carbs 39g | Fiber 3g | Sugars 25g | Protein 12g

85. Strawberry Banana Smoothie Refresh

Preparation Time: 5 Minutes | Total Time: 5 Minutes | Serves: 2

Ingredients:

- 1 frozen banana
- 1 fresh banana
- 1 cup Vanilla Bean Smoothie or vanilla kefir
- 1 cup sliced strawberries
- 1 to 2 teaspoons agave nectar

Directions:

1. Combine frozen and fresh bananas with Vanilla Bean Smoothie (or kefir) and strawberries in a blender, creating a fruity concoction.

2. Sweeten with agave nectar to taste, ensuring a perfect balance of flavors.

3. Pour the smoothie into two glasses for a vitamin-rich,

replenishing beverage ideal after any fitness routine.

Nutrition per serving: 200 Calories | Fat 1g | Sodium 40mg | Carbs 43g | Fiber 5g | Sugars 28g | Protein 8g

86. Blueberry Omega Shake Energizer

Preparation Time: 5 Minutes | Total Time: 5 Minutes | Serves: 1

Ingredients:

- 1 cup fresh blueberries
- ½ cup nonfat plain Greek yogurt
- ½ cup 100% blueberry juice
- 1 tablespoon Barlean's Pomegranate Blueberry Total Omega Swirl flax oil

Directions:

1. Blend blueberries, yogurt, and blueberry juice until smooth, infusing your shake with antioxidants.

2. Incorporate the omega swirl oil for an omega-3 fatty acids boost, blending until just combined.

3. Enjoy this nutrient-dense shake immediately, perfect for supporting recovery and overall well-being after strenuous activity.

Nutrition per serving: 270 Calories | Fat 6g | Saturated Fat 0.5g | Sodium 60mg | Carbs 45g | Fiber 4g | Sugars 32g | Protein 13g

87. Tropical Tempeh Smoothie Delight

Preparation Time: 5 Minutes | Total Time: 5 Minutes | Serves: 1

Ingredients:

- 2 ounces tempeh
- 1 cup 100% orange juice
- ½ cup frozen pineapple cubes
- 2 teaspoons coconut oil

Directions:

1. Combine tempeh, orange juice, pineapple, and coconut oil in a blender, creating a tropical-tasting, protein-rich smoothie.

2. Blend until creamy and smooth, ensuring the flavors meld together beautifully.

3. Serve this vibrant smoothie right away, offering a burst of energy and a hefty dose of vitamin C, essential for post-workout recovery.

Nutrition per serving: 320 Calories | Fat 12g | Saturated Fat 8g | Sodium 25mg | Carbs 46g | Fiber 2g | Sugars 28g | Protein 9g

88. Tart Cherry– Chia Kombucha

Preparation Time: 5 Minutes | Total Time: 15 Minutes | Serves: 1

Ingredients:

- ½ cup 100% tart cherry juice

- ½ cup GT's Enlightened Organic Raw Original Kombucha
- 1 tablespoon chia seeds

Directions:

1. Mix cherry juice, kombucha, and chia seeds in a glass, stirring well.
2. Allow the mixture to rest for 5-10 minutes for chia seeds to hydrate.
3. Enjoy fresh or keep chilled for up to 3-4 days.

Nutrition per serving: 150 Calories | Fat 5g | Saturated Fat 0.5g | Sodium 20mg | Carbs 25g | Fiber 5g | Sugars 14g | Protein 3g

89.   Black Cherry– Ginger Soda

Preparation Time: 5 Minutes | Total Time: 5 Minutes | Serves: 1

Ingredients:

- 1 cup frozen dark sweet cherries
- ½ cup black cherry seltzer or club soda
- ½ cup Ginger Beer

Directions:

1. Puree frozen cherries and seltzer until icy smooth in a blender.
2. In a glass, combine the blend with ginger beer, stirring gently.
3. Serve immediately to enjoy its refreshing taste.

Nutrition per serving: 140 Calories | Fat 0g | Sodium 0mg | Carbs 34g | Fiber 3g | Sugars 30g | Protein 1g

90.   Cherry Lime Kombucha Soda

Preparation Time: 2 Minutes | Total Time: 2 Minutes | Serves: 1

Ingredients:

- ½ cup Cherry Lime Fizz
- ¾ cup naturally flavored black cherry seltzer water

Directions:

1. Pour lime fizz into a glass, followed by the seltzer.
2. Stir gently to mix the bubbly goodness.
3. Sip immediately to savor its refreshing zest.

Nutrition per serving: 50 Calories | Fat 0g | Sodium 0mg | Carbs 13g | Fiber 2g | Sugars 10g | Protein <1g

91.   Chia Pudding Smoothie

Preparation Time: Overnight for Pudding + 5 Minutes for Smoothie | Total Time: Overnight + 5 Minutes | Serves: 2

Ingredients for Chia Pudding:

- 2 cups light almond milk or Homemade Almond Milk
- ½ cup chia seeds
- 1 tablespoon pure maple syrup

Ingredients for Smoothie:

- ½ cup low-fat or nonfat vanilla yogurt
- ½ teaspoon ground cinnamon

Directions:

1. Prepare chia pudding by mixing almond milk, chia seeds, and maple syrup. Refrigerate overnight until pudding consistency is achieved.

2. For the smoothie, blend 1½ cups chia pudding with yogurt and cinnamon until smooth.

3. Serve in glasses or store chilled for a quick breakfast or snack.

Nutrition per serving: 270 Calories | Fat 16g | Saturated Fat 2g | Sodium 135mg | Carbs 30g | Fiber 14g | Sugars 14g | Protein 10g

92. Creamy Watermelon Smoothie

Preparation Time: 5 Minutes | Total Time: 5 Minutes | Serves: 2

Ingredients:

- 3 cups cubed watermelon
- ½ cup low-fat or nonfat plain yogurt or Homemade Yogurt
- 8 ice cubes
- 1 to 2 teaspoons honey (optional)

Directions:

1. Blend watermelon, yogurt, and ice until smooth. Sweeten with honey if desired.

2. Divide between two glasses and enjoy a light, hydrating treat.

Nutrition per serving: 100 Calories | Fat 1g | Saturated Fat 0.5g | Sodium 40mg | Carbs 21g | Fiber <1g | Sugars 18g | Protein 4g

93. Green Chia Kefir Fusion

Preparation Time: 2 Minutes | Total Time: 2 Minutes | Serves: 1

Ingredients:

- 1 cup Traditional Plain Kefir
- 1 tablespoon chia seeds
- 1 teaspoon spirulina
- 1 teaspoon agave nectar

Directions:

1. In a glass, combine kefir, chia seeds, spirulina, and agave nectar. Stir well.

2. Savor the blend of probiotics, omega-3s, and superfoods in this nutrient-packed drink.

Nutrition per serving: 220 Calories | Fat 8g | Saturated Fat 2.5g | Sodium 240mg | Carbs 25g | Fiber 6g | Sugars 17g | Protein 19g

94. Honeydew Lime Refresher

Preparation Time: 5 Minutes | Total Time: 5 Minutes | Serves: 2

Ingredients:

- 1 cup cubed honeydew melon
- ½ cup low-fat or nonfat plain yogurt or Homemade Yogurt
- 1 tablespoon fresh Key lime juice
- 4 or 5 ice cubes

Directions:

1. Blend honeydew, yogurt, Key lime juice, and ice until silky smooth.

2. Distribute the smoothie into glasses for a revitalizing, low-calorie treat.

Nutrition per serving: 70 Calories | Fat 0g | Saturated Fat 0g | Sodium 40mg | Carbs 11g | Fiber <1g | Sugars 9g | Protein 6g

95. Macaroon Smoothie Luxe

Preparation Time: 5 Minutes | Total Time: 5 Minutes | Serves: 2

Ingredients:

- 1 cup So Delicious coconut milk beverage

- ¼ cup So Delicious unsweetened cultured coconut milk

- 1 tablespoon organic coconut palm sugar

- 4 or 5 ice cubes

- 1 tablespoon unsweetened coconut flakes, toasted

Directions:

1. Blend coconut milk, cultured coconut milk, sugar, and ice until perfectly smooth.

2. Toast coconut flakes in a skillet until golden, then sprinkle on top of the smoothie.

Nutrition per serving: 110 Calories | Fat 8g | Saturated Fat 7g | Sodium 10mg | Carbs 12g | Fiber 2g | Sugars 9g | Protein 0g

96. Watermelon Freeze Fizz

Preparation Time: 5 Minutes | Total Time: 5 Minutes | Serves: 1

Ingredients:

- 2 cups cubed watermelon

- 6 ice cubes

- 1 cup naturally flavored black cherry seltzer

- ¼ cup Coconut Water Kefir

Directions:

1. Blend watermelon and ice until smooth. Add a splash of water if needed for easier blending.

2. Pour into a glass, top with black cherry seltzer and Coconut Water Kefir, and gently mix.

3. Serve this luscious lycopene-loaded freeze for a hydrating, probiotic punch.

Nutrition per serving: 140 Calories | Fat 0.5g | Saturated Fat 0g | Sodium 75mg | Carbs 35g | Fiber 3g | Sugars 27g | Protein 2g

97. Honey Pear Shake Delight

Preparation Time: 5 Minutes | Total Time: 5 Minutes | Serves: 2

Ingredients:

- 2 ripe Bartlett pears, cored

- ½ cup low-fat or nonfat buttermilk

- ¼ cup water

- 2 teaspoons honey

Directions:

1. Blend pears, buttermilk, water, and honey until silky and perfectly smooth.

2. If needed, adjust thickness with more water or ice, according to preference.

3. Serve this light, fiber-rich shake for a quick, refreshing snack or breakfast boost.

Nutrition per serving: 140 Calories | Fat 1.5g | Saturated Fat 1g | Cholesterol <5mg | Sodium 55mg | Carbs 31g | Fiber 4g | Sugars 23g | Protein 3g

98. Jose Grabowski Pickle Shot

Prep & Total Time: 5 Minutes | Serves: 2

Ingredients:

- 1 large dill pickle (e.g., Bubbies Pure Kosher Dills), halved crosswise

- 2 ounces tequila

Directions:

1. Use a melon baller to hollow out each pickle half into a shot glass.

2. Pour tequila into each pickle and toast to tradition. Follow the tequila shot with a pickle chaser for a salty crunch.

Nutrition per serving: 90 Calories | Sodium 870mg | Carbs 3g

99. Ginger Bellini Peach Twist

Prep & Total Time: 10 Minutes | Serves: 2

Ingredients:

- 1 cup frozen peaches

- 1 cup water

- 1 cup ginger beer

- 2 fresh peach slices for garnish

Directions:

1. Blend frozen peaches and water until smooth.

2. Pour into glasses, stir in ginger beer, and garnish with peach slices.

Nutrition per serving: 80 Calories | Carbs 20g | Vitamin C 10%

100. Apple Ginger Soda Refresh

Prep & Total Time: 5 Minutes | Serves: 1

Ingredients:

- 4 or 5 ice cubes

- ½ cup apple cider

- ½ cup ginger beer

Directions:

1. Combine ice, cider, and ginger beer in a glass for a fizzy treat.

Nutrition per serving: 110 Calories | Carbs 26g | Vitamin C 50%

101. Kombucha Root Beer Float

Prep & Total Time: 5 Minutes | Serves: 1

Ingredients:

- ½ cup original kombucha
- ¼ teaspoon root beer extract
- ½ cup vanilla frozen yogurt

Directions:

1. Mix kombucha with root beer extract, then top with vanilla frozen yogurt.

2. Savor this innovative twist on the classic float, brimming with probiotic flair.

Nutrition per serving: 120 Calories | Sodium 70mg | Carbs 24g | Protein 4g

PART 3 EXERCISE

The fun Gutsy Challenge

Feeling sluggish, bloated, or just not quite yourself? It's time to show your gut some love! The Gutsy Challenge is a 20-question test of how well you know the secrets to a happy, healthy digestive system. Along the way, you'll discover tips, tricks, and the science behind a healthy gut.

Instructions:

1. Read each question carefully.

2. Choose the answer you think is best.

3. Don't worry if you aren't sure – this is about learning!

4. At the end, check your answers and see what your gut health knowledge is like.

Let's get started!

Question 1: Which of these contributes to an unhealthy gut?

- A) Regular exercise

- B) Eating plenty of fruits and vegetables

- C) Frequently consuming processed foods

- D) Getting enough sleep

Question 2: The Gut C.A.R.E. program is made up of these steps:

- A) Create, Activate, Repair, Expand

- B) Cook, Analyze, Rethink, Educate

- C) Cleanse, Activate, Restore, Enhance

- D) Cravings, Appetite, Reduce, Exercise

Question 3: True or False: Your gut only affects your digestion.

Question 4: Which of these is NOT a symptom of an unhappy gut?

- A) Bloating and gas

- B) Frequent headaches

- C) Strong, healthy hair

- D) Mood swings

Question 5: During the "Cleanse" phase of the Gut C.A.R.E. program, what do you cut out of your diet?

- A) Foods you might be sensitive to, like gluten and dairy
- B) All carbohydrates
- C) Anything that tastes good
- D) Red meat and poultry

Question 6: What helps your body digest food, taking pressure off your gut?

- A) Digestive enzymes
- B) Multivitamins
- C) Extra servings of dessert
- D) Spicy foods

Question 7: Friendly bacteria that live in your gut are called:

- A) Probiotics
- B) Parasites
- C) Enzymes
- D) Microbes

Question 8: True or False: Your gut health can impact your mood and mental wellbeing.

Question 9: What can help heal the lining of your gut?

- A) L-glutamine
- B) Coffee
- C) Sugar
- D) Alcohol

Question 10: The 15-Day Gut Cleanse focuses on:

- A) Eating as little food as possible
- B) Nourishing foods and gut-supportive habits
- C) Only drinking juice
- D) Cutting out all fruits and vegetables

Question 11: Which type of food supports the good bacteria in your gut?

- A) Probiotic
- B) Prebiotic

- C) Processed
- D) Pickled

Question 12: Which drink is a great way to get gut-friendly probiotics?

- A) Kefir
- B) Soda
- C) Sports drink
- D) Sweetened iced tea

Question 13: Why does the Gut C.A.R.E. program include a focus on reducing stress?

- A) Stress helps our gut bacteria thrive
- B) Stress has no impact on the gut
- C) Stress can disrupt digestion and gut health
- D) Stress helps us eat healthier

Question 14: How does drinking enough water help your gut function?

- A) It aids in digestion and regularity
- B) It dehydrates your gut
- C) It makes you crave sugary drinks
- D) It has no effect on the digestive system

Question 15: What's a sign that you may be experiencing detox symptoms during a cleanse?

- A) A slight headache
- B) Feeling super energetic
- C) Clear thinking
- D) No bloating or gas

Questions 16-20: Match these gut-healthy foods with their benefits:

A) Fermented yogurt * **B)** Chia seeds * **C)** Oatmeal * **D)** Berries * **E)** Salmon

1. Packed with healthy fats for gut health
2. Rich in antioxidants and fiber
3. Excellent source of prebiotics
4. Provides probiotics for a thriving gut

5. Good source of soluble fiber

Answers and Explanations to the Quiz

1. **C** (Frequently consuming processed foods)

2. **C** (Cleanse, Activate, Restore, Enhance)

3. **False** (Your gut influences many systems in your body)

4. **C** (Strong, healthy hair)

5. **A** (Foods you might be sensitive to)

6. **A** (Digive enzymes)

7. **A** (Probiotics)

8. **True**

9. **A** (L-glutamine)

10. **B** (Nourishing foods and gut-supportive habits)

11. **B** (Prebiotic)

12. **A** (Kefir)

13. **C** (Stress can disrupt digestion and gut health)

14. **A** (It aids in digestion and regularity)

15. **A** (A slight headache)

16. **A - 4**

17. **B - 2**

18. **C - 3**

19. **D - 2**

20. **E - 1**

Explanations

- **Processed foods:** Often lack fiber, have unhealthy fats, and are high in sugar – bad news for your gut.

- **Gut health and your brain:** There's a strong connection (the gut-brain axis)!

- **Symptoms of an unhappy gut:** Don't dismiss bloating, mood swings, or headaches – your gut might be trying to tell you something.

- **Detox symptoms:** Common during cleanses as your body adjusts.

PART 4: SUPPORTING YOUR GUT THROUGH LIFESTYLE PRACTICES

CHAPTER 10

Exercise, Mental Well-being, skin and Gut Health
"Those who think they have no time for bodily exercise will sooner or later have to find time for illness." - Edward Stanley

They tell you to work out to look better, lose weight, to have a strong heart. But there's a whole hidden side to exercise that no one at the gym is talking about, a secret that could completely transform your life. The truth is, getting your body moving isn't just about how you look – it's about your mental health, your mood, and yes, even the health of your gut. And if you mess this up, the consequences aren't just a few extra pounds; we're talking about a total meltdown from the inside out.

The Mind-Gut-Muscle Connection

Imagine you are stressed and anxious, and the world feels heavy. What's your first instinct? For many of us, it's to curl up on the couch and numb those feelings. But what if I told you the best medicine might be the one thing you feel least like doing... lacing up those sneakers and getting your sweat on?

Here's the breakdown:

- **Your Brain on Exercise:** When you workout, your body unleashes a cocktail of feel-good chemicals. Endorphins, nature's painkiller...you've heard of those, right? But it doesn't stop there. Exercise also boosts dopamine (your reward chemical), and serotonin (the mood stabilizer), and lowers cortisol (the stress hormone). Basically, it's a natural mood-boosting, stress-busting, anxiety-taming potion.

- **Your Gut's Happy Dance:** Remember that gut microbiome, the trillions of little critters influencing your whole body? Well, exercise changes the game for them. Research shows that regular physical activity increases the diversity and number of those "good bacteria." This strengthens your gut-brain connection and has a ripple effect throughout your entire system.

- **The Two-Way Street:** That gut-brain connection isn't a one-way deal, though. A healthy gut with a balanced microbiome sends its own "chill out" signals to your brain, further reducing anxiety and improving your overall mood. It's a beautiful harmony that makes the struggle seem less overwhelming.

The Science Behind Mental Well-being and Gut Health

I know, it sounds a bit too good to be true. But check this out:

- **Depression Destroyer:** Studies show that regular exercise can be as effective as antidepressant medication for mild to moderate depression. And guess what? No nasty side effects with this treatment!

- **Anxiety Eraser:** Feeling jittery and on edge? Exercise is proven to significantly reduce symptoms of anxiety disorders, sometimes working better than certain medications.

- **Gut Health Champion:** Researchers are finding that exercise actually alters the types of bacteria living in your gut, favoring the beneficial ones that boost immunity, and metabolism, and even fight inflammation.

- **Stress Shield:** Ever notice how a stressful day can totally wreck your digestive system? Exercise builds resilience. It helps your body manage stress more effectively, which also benefits those good gut bugs.

- **Brain Fog No More:** Regular workouts improve mental clarity, focus, and memory. You know that brain fog weighing you down? Consider exercising your mental broom sweeping it away.

BUT...There's a Catch

- **Type Matters:** Not all exercise is created equal for optimal mental and gut health. While any movement has some benefits, aim for:

  - Moderate-intensity cardio: Think brisk walks, jogging, swimming, dancing – get that heart pumping for at least 30 minutes most days.

  - Strength training: Lifting weights a few days a week is key for building muscle and boosting your metabolism.

- Mind-Body Connection: Activities like yoga and tai chi combine movement with mindfulness for an extra dose of stress relief.

- **Overdoing It is Bad News:** You might think "more is better" applies here, but not so fast! Pushing yourself way too hard, to the point of exhaustion, can actually worsen your mood, increase stress hormones, and mess with your gut bacteria in the wrong way.

- **Food Still Matters**: All those exercise benefits get magnified with a healthy diet. Eating junk and expecting workouts to magically fix everything is a recipe for disappointment.

How does this change everything?

This information isn't some feel-good fluff. It has the power to transform your life:

- **Finding Motivation When Times Are Tough:** Depression, and anxiety, make just getting out of bed an epic battle. But knowing exercise can ease those very symptoms gives you a powerful reason to push through. It's not about willpower, it's about having a tool that works.

- **Ditching the Quick Fixes:** Pills, booze, self-medicating with unhealthy habits...those offer temporary relief and often worsen the problem down the line. Exercise offers a sustainable, healthy path to feeling better.

- **Taking Control:** If you've felt powerless over your mood or your health, this is a game-changer. You can actively improve your well-being, both physically and mentally, with every workout. That's empowering!

A Note of Caution

If you're new to exercise, have any health conditions, or are dealing with severe mental health issues, please consult your doctor before starting any new program. Exercise is a powerful medicine, but it needs to be personalized for your needs!

The Gut-Skin Connection

Think those breakouts, wrinkles, and dullness are just bad luck or genetics? Think again. The food industry bombards you with junk disguised as delicious, and Big Pharma peddles quick-fix creams that never address the actual issue. They don't want you to realize the power you hold over your complexion – power that starts with healing your gut. This isn't just about skincare; this is about unlocking the radiant, healthy skin you were always meant to have.

Your Skin: A Mirror of Your Gut

Your skin isn't just a pretty covering; it's your body's largest organ and a direct reflection of what's happening on the inside. When your gut is a war zone, your skin shows it:

- **Acne: Breakouts That Won't Quit:** Gut inflammation triggers a domino effect that leads to oily skin, clogged pores, and angry pimples you hate.

- **Eczema, Psoriasis, Rosacea: The Inflammation Link** A messed-up gut microbiome sets your entire body's immune system on high alert, making inflammatory skin conditions worse.

- **Dry, Dull Skin:** When your gut can't properly absorb nutrients, your skin is deprived of the vital building blocks it needs to stay hydrated and glowing.

- **Accelerated Aging:** Your gut produces collagen-boosting compounds. When it's out of whack, say hello to premature wrinkles and sagging.

How Does Your Gut Mess Up Your Skin?

Here's a breakdown of the not-so-pretty cycle:

1. **Gut Imbalance is Born:** Processed foods, sugar overload, stress, medications...these things wreak havoc on your delicate gut microbiome. Bad bacteria start to take over.

2. **Dripping Gut: The Gateway to Trouble** Your gut lining is supposed to be selectively permeable – letting good stuff in, and keeping the bad stuff out. But gut imbalance damages this lining, making it "leaky."

3. **Toxins and Inflammation Run Wild:** When food particles and bacteria slip through your leaky gut, your immune system goes haywire. Chronic, body-wide inflammation is the result.

4. **Your Skin Pays the Price:** This inflammation messes with hormone balance, oil production, and skin cell renewal, leading to acne, dryness, and premature aging. Plus, impaired nutrient absorption leaves your skin starving.

The Science Behind the Madness

This isn't some new-age theory, there's solid research confirming the gut-skin connection:

- **Inflammatory Skin Conditions:** Studies consistently show that people with conditions like acne, psoriasis, and eczema have higher rates of intestinal problems like leaky gut and bacterial imbalance.

- **Probiotics Improve Skin Health:** Several trials demonstrate that taking specific probiotic strains can significantly reduce acne severity and improve markers of skin hydration and elasticity.

- **Diet Matters:** A clean, whole-food diet nourishes your gut AND your skin, while junk food fuels the fire that leads to both gut distress and skin woes.

The Gut-Skin SOS: What Can You Do?

Remember the power you hold? It's time to reclaim it! Here's how to support your gut and transform your skin:

- **Ditch the Destroyers:**
  - Processed foods: They're gut bacteria rocket fuel...of the bad kind.
  - Refined Sugar: Your gut microbiome hates it, and your skin will show it.
  - Excessive Alcohol: Impairs gut lining and feeds harmful bacteria.
  - Unnecessary Medications: Talk to your doctor about how essential those antibiotics or other regular meds are.

- **Load Up on Gut-Loving Goodness:**

- Fermented Foods: Yogurt, kimchi, sauerkraut – natural sources of probiotics.

- Prebiotic-Rich Foods: Think garlic, onions, bananas, oats – feed those good bacteria.

- Fiber Powerhouse: Whole fruits, veggies, legumes, nuts, seeds – essential for healthy digestion and a happy gut microbiome.

- Quality Probiotic Supplement: Ask your doctor or a functional medicine practitioner for recommendations based on your specific needs.

Additional Skin Support:

While gut healing is key, you can boost things further:

- **Gentle Cleansing:** Harsh cleansers strip your skin, making it more vulnerable.

- **Hydration, Hydration, Hydration:** Water is your skin's BFF! Topical hyaluronic acid serums also help.

- **Stress Management:** Meditation, yoga, spending time in nature – your gut AND skin benefit from finding your zen.

CHAPTER 11

Probiotics and Prebiotics: Understanding the Differences

"The doctor of the future will no longer treat the human frame with drugs, but rather will cure and prevent disease with nutrition." – Thomas Edison

Probiotics vs. Prebiotics: What's the Difference?

Okay, picture your gut like a messy, overgrown garden. It's got weeds, some withered plants, and maybe a few flowers struggling to survive. Here's the deal:

- **Probiotics: The Good Seeds.** Probiotics are live bacteria and yeasts - the good guys! Taking a probiotic is like scattering beneficial seeds throughout your messed-up garden. These new guys compete with the weeds (the harmful bacteria that make you feel awful), restoring balance and helping those struggling flowers flourish.

- **Prebiotics: The Super-Fertilizer.** Prebiotics are indigestible fibers that feed those good bacteria you just planted. Think of it like showering your garden with the richest fertilizer, giving the good seeds the fuel they need to colonize and dominate, crowding out those nasty weeds long-term.

Why These Duo Matters

Probiotics and prebiotics aren't "nice to have"; they're essential for optimal health. Here's the catch: modern life is constantly bombarding your gut:

- **Processed junk food:** Full of chemicals and empty calories, starving your good bacteria.

- **Antibiotics:** These kill off harmful bacteria when you're sick, but they wipe out the good guys too.

- **Stress:** It messes with EVERYTHING, including your gut health.

The result? An overgrown, chaotic mess down there. One where the bad guys thrive, leading to:

- **Digestive Havoc:** Bloating, gas, IBS...the kind of symptoms that make you avoid social situations.

- **Weakened Immunity:** Your gut is where most of your immune system lives. Wreck it, and you're a walking target for every bug.

- **Stubborn Weight Gain:** Gut bacteria play a HUGE role in how your body uses energy and stores fat. Bad gut = bad metabolism.

- **Mental Fog:** Gut bacteria make neurotransmitters that affect your mood, focus, and even anxiety.

Long-term gut imbalance is linked to stuff you really don't want: autoimmune diseases, heart problems, and even certain cancers. This is why understanding probiotics and prebiotics isn't a cute health trend – it's about defending yourself from future misery!

Important Info on Probiotics

Let's get a bit more specific on these "good seeds":

- **Different Strains Matter:** Not all probiotics are created equal! Think of Lactobacillus as a helpful gardener, while Bifidobacterium is the master weed-killer. Each strain offers unique benefits.

- **Temporary Tenants:** Most probiotics don't permanently take up residence in your gut. You need continued reinforcement for lasting results.

- **The Science:** Solid evidence for probiotics helping with:

  o Diarrhea (especially after antibiotics)
  o IBS symptoms
  o Certain skin conditions (like eczema)
  o May protect against some infections

Prebiotics: The Silent Heroes

These special fibers might not get as much hype as probiotics, but they are the key to long-term gut transformation:

- **The Fuel Good Bacteria Crave:** Specific prebiotics nourish specific strains. Think of it like targeted fertilizing to optimize your gut's ecosystem.

- **Types to Look For:**
  - Inulin
  - Fructooligosaccharides (FOS)
  - Galactooligosaccharides (GOS)
- **The Science:** Research suggests prebiotics may help with:
  - Improved mineral absorption (like calcium for strong bones)
  - Better blood sugar control
  - Reduced gut inflammation

The Power of Probiotics & Prebiotics in the real-world

I could fill a book with the scientific studies backing all of this (and hey, maybe I will someday). But here's the thing you need to understand:

- **Gut Transformation = Whole Body Transformation:** Better digestion, stronger immunity, clearer thinking, increased energy... all possible when you get your gut right.

- **Not a Substitute for Healthy Living:** These are incredibly powerful tools, but they can't magically undo the damage from an otherwise terrible lifestyle.

- **Everyone's Gut is Unique:** What works wonders for your friend might be meh for you. Some experimentation is part of the journey.

- **This is the REAL Healthcare:** Forget symptom masking with pills. True disease prevention starts with nurturing your gut's intricate balance.

The Role of Supplements and Other Gut-Supporting Products

They want you hooked on pills, potions, and fad diets designed to fail. They want you confused, frustrated, and convinced that being bloated and miserable is just "how it is" past a certain age. But they're not telling you the whole story. Sometimes, your gut needs a little extra help to get back on track. That's where quality supplements and other gut-supporting tools come in – but you have to know what actually works and what's just a waste of your hard-earned cash. Let's break it down.

Understanding Supplements: They're Not All Created Equal

The supplement industry is like the Wild West. Some brands are amazing, others are peddling snake oil in a fancy bottle. Here's the truth bomb: Not all supplements are necessary, and even the good ones won't magically undo a terrible diet and other unhealthy habits.

But, when used strategically, the right supplements can give your gut the healing boost it craves, especially when you're dealing with those annoying gut problems that just won't quit.

Supplements with Potential Gut Benefits

- **Probiotics:** We've hammered this one home, but good-quality probiotic supplements can restore balance and ease various digestive woes. Choose strains backed by research for your specific concerns.

- **Prebiotics:** If you struggle to get enough prebiotic-rich food in your diet, supplementing can encourage the growth of your resident good bacteria friends.

- **Digestive Enzymes:** These guys help your body break down food properly. Beneficial if you experience constant uncomfortable gas and bloating, especially after meals.

- **L-Glutamine:** This amino acid might help repair a leaky gut lining, potentially easing IBS, bloating, and food allergies. It's a promising area of research!

- **Herbal Remedies:** Things like ginger, peppermint, and chamomile have been used for centuries to soothe upset stomachs. But talk to your doctor, especially if you take medication, as they can interact.

Addressing Common Gut Concerns – Beyond the Basics

Let's be real; most of us have experienced these gut nightmares:

- **Bloating:** Feeling like a pufferfish after eating? A combo of probiotic supplements, digestive enzymes, and reducing common food triggers (dairy, gluten, etc.) could be your ticket to relief.

- **Constipation:** Magnesium supplements can help with the, ahem, movement of things. Fiber supplements like psyllium husk also work wonders, but drink tons of water along with them!

- **Diarrhea:** While it's important to see a doctor to rule out anything serious, probiotics designed for diarrhea can help, along with a temporarily bland diet to let your gut rest.

- **Leaky Gut:** This buzzword gets thrown around a lot, and there's debate on its exact definition. But some supplements, like L-glutamine, zinc, and bone broth, might help strengthen your intestinal lining.

Other Gut-Supporting Products to Consider

- **Gut-Healing Powders:** Many contain combos of prebiotics, probiotics, L-glutamine, and soothing ingredients for when your gut is in full-on revolt.

- **Natural Laxatives:** Senna or stimulant laxatives are not for long-term use, but in a constipation emergency, they can be a temporary solution. Always talk to your doctor.

- **Stress-Management Tools:** Yup, stress messes with your gut! Meditation apps, soothing teas, or even a walk in nature can make a surprising difference.

The Scientific Exposé

While many natural remedies show promise, the research on gut health supplements is still evolving. Here's the deal:

- **Not One-Size-Fits-All:** What works for your friend's IBS might not help you at all. Experimentation and listening to your body is key.

- **Talk To A Pro:** Doctors specializing in functional medicine are often better positioned to recommend specific supplements than your regular GP who might not be up on the latest gut health research.

- **The Food Foundation:** Supplements won't fix everything. A gut-healthy diet rich in whole foods and fiber is still a non-negotiable base.

WARNING SIGNS: When to Skip Supplements & See a Doctor

- **Constant, Severe Pain:** Don't self-diagnose with supplements. Rule out serious issues first!

- **Blood in Stool:** Black, tarry, or bright red – get to a doctor ASAP.

- **Sudden, Unexplained Weight Loss:** This is never a good sign, supplements won't help.

- **Chronic Conditions:** Heart disease, diabetes, autoimmune diseases – always involve your doctor in your supplement plan.

Red Flags: When to Seek Help

Your gut isn't just about poop. Think of it as your body's internal alarm system, whispering (or sometimes SCREAMING) when something's seriously off. Sadly, most of us have been trained to ignore those signals, popping pills for the symptoms while the root problem festers. But guess what? Your body's not giving up on you. It's going to keep throwing up those red flags until you pay attention. Learning to spot them is the first step to taking control of your health – and I'm here to spill the beans.

Red Flags That Mean "GET HELP...NOW!"

These aren't your everyday digestive grumbles. Don't brush them off as "just stress" or assume they'll go away on their own:

- **Blood in Your Stool:** Whether bright red, dark, tarry, or microscopic (only found through a test), blood where it shouldn't be is a major red flag. Could be anything from minor hemorrhoids to serious stuff like ulcers, inflammatory bowel disease, or even cancer. Don't wait, get checked.

- **Sudden, Severe Weight Loss:** Dropped a few pounds due to better eating? Great! Dropping weight rapidly without trying is a whole different story. It could point to digestive problems preventing absorption, infections, and even hidden cancers.

- **Constant Diarrhea or Constipation:** We all have "off" days, but when major swings in bowel habits become your new normal for weeks on end, it's time for answers. Persistent gut changes can signal infections, bowel diseases, or issues with organs like your thyroid.

- **Intense Abdominal Pain:** Mild cramps are one thing, but sudden onset, severe pain that makes you double over or disrupts your life is never normal. It could be an obstructed bowel, appendicitis, gallbladder problems, or a whole host of serious issues.

- **Fever, Vomiting Along With Gut Trouble:** This combo isn't just a nasty stomach bug. It might mean a serious infection, food poisoning, or a flare-up of an underlying gut disease. When things get violent, get seen.

- **Pain That Changes Dramatically:** Did that ache suddenly shift locations? Did it go from dull to sharp? That's a warning sign that something could be getting worse quickly, like an appendix about to burst.

Chronic Red Flags: Less Urgent, Still Important

These might be easier to dismiss at first, but they're sabotaging your quality of life. They're strong clues that your gut health is out of whack and needs to be addressed ASAP:

- **Gas and Bloating That Won't Quit:** It's not just embarrassing; constant bloating can be crazily uncomfortable and point to food intolerances, imbalances in your gut bacteria, conditions like SIBO (small intestinal bacterial overgrowth), and more.

- **Heartburn or Reflux That Doesn't Respond:** Over-the-counter meds giving you no relief? That burning feeling and acid creeping up your throat can damage your esophagus over time, and sometimes it's a sign of something unexpected, like an H. pylori infection.

- **Skin Problems That Defy Treatment:** Chronic acne, eczema, psoriasis...it might not seem gut-related, but inflammation in the gut often shows up on your skin. Don't just cover it up; get to the root cause.

- **Unstoppable Fatigue:** If you're sleeping enough but still dragging, your gut might be to blame. Poor nutrient absorption, chronic inflammation, and gut problems throw your whole system out of balance.

- **Intense Food Cravings:** Can't stop reaching for sugar and junk? This could be a sign of bad bacteria hijacking your brain and manipulating you for your survival. Creepy, but true.

- **Brain Fog, Depression, Anxiety:** Your gut produces a ton of neurotransmitters that impact your mood. An unhappy gut often means an unhappy mind and chronic issues can worsen mental health conditions you already struggle with.

Why You Shouldn't Just Self-Diagnose

I know, Dr. Google is tempting. But here's the problem: symptoms overlap a lot. Bloating could be a simple food sensitivity or something more serious. A gut problem can even mimic symptoms of heart disease! A proper diagnosis is crucial for getting the right treatment and avoiding unnecessary worry.

What to Expect From a Doctor's Visit

- **Thorough History:** Be prepared to discuss everything from bowel habits to medications to your diet and stress levels. Honesty is key here!

- **Physical Exam:** They'll likely check your abdomen for tenderness, masses, or any abnormalities.

- **Tests:** The fun part (not). Could involve bloodwork, stool samples, imaging (like ultrasounds, CT scans), or procedures like a colonoscopy. Don't be scared, these tests are how we get answers.

Take good care of yourself, and don't wait until you have to be admitted to the hospital before you take things seriously, your body is the only temple you can live in, TAKE GOOD CARE OF IT!

Juliet's Experience

My name is Juliet and I have a beautiful healthy boy named Justin whom I almost lost.

The screaming was unbearable. Justin, my usually cheerful little boy, was in severe pain, his tiny body wracked with sobs. I held him close, guilt and fear washing over me. As doctors poked and prodded, my mind raced – what had I done wrong? Was this my fault?

The diagnosis – a blocked intestine caused by a blood clot – was terrifying and confusing. Justin, so full of life, was suddenly hooked up to machines, his future uncertain. Days turned into weeks, spent in the sterile confines of the hospital. When he was finally discharged on blood thinners, I was relieved but terrified. How would we manage this? Would he ever be a normal kid?

Justin surprised us all. With the resilience of childhood, he bounced back. But there were lingering issues…bloating, tummy aches, and a growing fear of food. Mealtimes became battles, and my heart ached to see my once-adventurous eater turn picky and anxious.

Desperate for answers, I stumbled upon information about gut health and its connection to overall well-being by Barbara O'Neill. It was like a lightbulb went off. Jude's intense medical treatment had likely wreaked havoc on his delicate gut microbiome. Could this explain the ongoing problems, the lingering anxieties?

Inspired by Barbara O'Neill's Cleansing teachings, I revamped our diet. Processed snacks were replaced with whole fruits and vegetables. We discovered the power of fermented foods – yogurt became a staple, kimchi a curious adventure. Instead of sugary treats, we experimented with naturally sweet energy bites packed with prebiotic-rich goodness.

The change wasn't always easy. Justin missed his familiar favorites. But gradually, something shifted. The bloating subsided, and his energy returned. The picky eating lessened as his gut began to heal. And the biggest transformation? The anxiety around food began to lift. Mealtimes became less stressful, laughter replaced tears.

Seeing Justin truly enjoy food again was a revelation. More importantly, it felt like we were giving him a chance at a normal, healthy childhood, not defined by his earlier medical trauma. His journey also revealed a passion for nutrition and the incredible power of food as medicine.

Of course, this isn't a fairy-tale cure. Consulting with Justin's doctors remains essential. Yet, the empowerment of taking control, of actively nurturing his gut health, has made a world of difference.

Today, Justin is a thriving, adventurous boy. He still loves the occasional slice of pizza, but he also reaches for a handful of berries or a homemade smoothie with a grin. He knows that what he eats makes his tummy feel good and that knowledge fuels healthy choices.

Juliet's story of her son Justin is a reminder of the incredible resilience of the human body, the interconnectedness of our physical and mental well-being, and the power of a mother determined to support her child's health in any way she can.

CONCLUSION

Strategy to Maintain a Healthy Gut Throughout Your Life

"The groundwork of all happiness is good health." – Leigh Hunt

Okay, by now, the message should be loud and clear: your gut isn't just about poop, and neglect comes at a serious cost. This 15-Day Cleanse is your kick-start, the eye-opening experience that shows you what a balanced gut feels like. But the real victory comes in making this a lasting lifestyle shift, not just a quick fix.

Let's face it, life happens. Parties, vacations, stressful weeks...you can't be perfect all the time. So how do we keep our gut health on track long-term without turning them into obsessive health nuts? Here's the deal:

- **The 80/20 Rule:** Focus on nourishing, gut-friendly choices most of the time. Then, when those occasional indulgences pop up, enjoy them without guilt, and get back on track afterward.

- **Listen to Your Body:** Did that pizza bloat you for days? Did eating more fiber finally clear things up? Your body is giving you constant feedback; pay attention and adjust accordingly.

- **Mind Over Matter:** Stress wreaks havoc on your gut. Find stress-busting techniques that work for you – exercise, meditation, or even just a 5-minute deep breathing session can help.

- **Sleep is Sacred:** Aim for those 7-8 hours. While you snooze, your body (and your gut!) are busy repairing and resetting.

- **Movement is Medicine:** Doesn't have to be the gym if that's not your thing. Walks, dancing, whatever gets you moving consistently boosts gut health.

Specific Strategies to Keep in Your Toolbox:

- **Probiotic Power:** Yogurt, fermented foods, or a quality supplement can be your daily gut guardians.

- **Prebiotic Fuel:** Prioritize those gut-loving fibers from fruits, veggies, and whole grains.

- **Hydration Station:** Water is essential for digestion and overall health. Aim for those classic 8 glasses a day, or more if you're active.

- **Manage Food Sensitivities:** Common triggers like gluten or dairy can cause gut chaos in some people. If something consistently bothers you stop having it.

- **The Supplement Question:** A good multivitamin can fill in nutritional gaps, and extra magnesium can help with regularity. But always check with your doctor before starting anything new.

The Big-Picture Mindset Shifts

Your gut is part of an interconnected system. Here's the thinking that'll keep you winning long-term:

- **Food as Medicine:** Skip the fads, and focus on real, whole foods as the foundation of your diet. Processed junk is the enemy, plain and simple.

- **Slow Down:** Chew thoroughly, eat mindfully. Digestion starts in the mouth, and savoring your food is good for the gut and the soul.

- **Tune In:** Did that meal make you feel amazing or sluggish? Your gut is trying to tell you something, so don't ignore it!

- **Progress, not Perfection:** Every little positive change counts and consistency beats the occasional super-healthy day followed by a junk-food binge.

This Isn't Just About Looking Better (Though You Probably Will!)

This is about feeling energized, dodging illness, and protecting yourself from chronic diseases down the road. Remember, that food industry and Big Pharma...they profit from you staying sick and confused. Knowledge is your weapon, and making your gut health a priority is how you take back the power.

This journey is uniquely yours. Some things will work better for you than others. But the commitment to learning, experimenting, and prioritizing this aspect of your health?

That's transformative. So go forth, my friend, armed with your newfound gut-health knowledge. This isn't the end; it's just the beginning!

Additional Resources and References

Trustworthy Resources: Where to Get the Good Stuff

We're aiming for credible, science-backed info, not random blogs pushing miracle cures.

1. **Reputable Organizations**

   o **The American Gastroenterological Association (AGA):** (https://gastro.org/) – Gut health guidelines, patient education, and the latest research.

   o **International Foundation for Gastrointestinal Disorders (IFFGD):** (https://iffgd.org/)– Fact sheets, diet tips, dedicated to digestive health.

   o **National Institutes of Health (NIH), Office of Dietary Supplements:** (https://ods.od.nih.gov/) – In-depth scientific info on probiotics, prebiotics, and other supplements.

   o **Center for Human Microbiome Studies at Stanford Medicine:** ([invalid URL removed]) – Cutting-edge research on your gut's inhabitants.

   o **World Gastroenterology Organisation (WGO):** (https://www.worldgastroenterology.org/) – Global resources, practice guidelines for digestive health professionals.

2. **Highly Respected Doctors & Researchers**

   o **Dr. Robynne Chutkan:** Author of "Gutbliss" and "The Microbiome Solution" (https://gutbliss.com/)

   o **Dr. Alessio Fasano:** Microbiome and celiac disease expert at Harvard Medical School ([invalid URL removed])

   o **Dr. Emeran Mayer:** Author of "The Mind-Gut Connection", UCLA researcher on brain-gut interactions (https://emeranmayer.com/)

   o **Dr. Mark Pimentel:** Expert on IBS and SIBO, Director of the GI Motility Program at Cedars-Sinai ([invalid URL removed])

3. **Scientific Journals (for those who want to go DEEP)**

   o **Gut:** (https://gut.bmj.com/) – Top-notch research on all things gastrointestinal

   o **Nature Reviews Gastroenterology & Hepatology:** (https://www.nature.com/nrgastro/) – Reviews of recent developments, clinical implications

   o **The American Journal of Clinical Nutrition:** (https://academic.oup.com/ajcn) – Often covers gut microbiome and its relation to nutrition

   o **Beneficial Microbes:** ([[invalid URL removed]]) – Focuses on the good guys, probiotics and their potential

   o **Neurogastroenterology & Motility:** (https://onlinelibrary.wiley.com/journal/13652982) – Where the brain-gut connection gets technical

4. **Informative Books (Beyond This One, Of Course!)**

   o **10% Human by Alanna Collen:** Delves into the whole microbiome picture, not just your gut.

   o **The Gut Makeover by Jeannette Hyde:** Practical 4-week plan based on gut health principles.

   o **Fiber Fueled by Dr. Will Bulsiewicz:** Plant-based approach, great for prebiotic enthusiasts.

   o **I Contain Multitudes by Ed Yong:** Beautifully written exploration of the microbial world within us.

5. **Reliable Websites and Blogs**

   o **Precision Nutrition:** (https://www.precisionnutrition.com/) - Evidence-based info, debunks myths.

   o **The Food Medic by Dr. Hazel Wallace:** (https://thefoodmedic.co.uk/) – Gut health focus, recipes with a UK-slant.

- o **Abbey's Kitchen:** (https://abbeyskitchen.com/) – Tons of gut-friendly recipes, focus on real food.

- o **NutritionFacts.org:** (https://nutritionfacts.org/) – Evidence-based summaries of studies, search their gut-related videos.

Even credible sources can change over time with new research. Be a critical thinker! Look for recent dates, and citations of peer-reviewed studies, and avoid sites with overly sales language.

9 781963 674217